BRO, SHE'S PREGNANT
Dad's week by week pregnancy guide

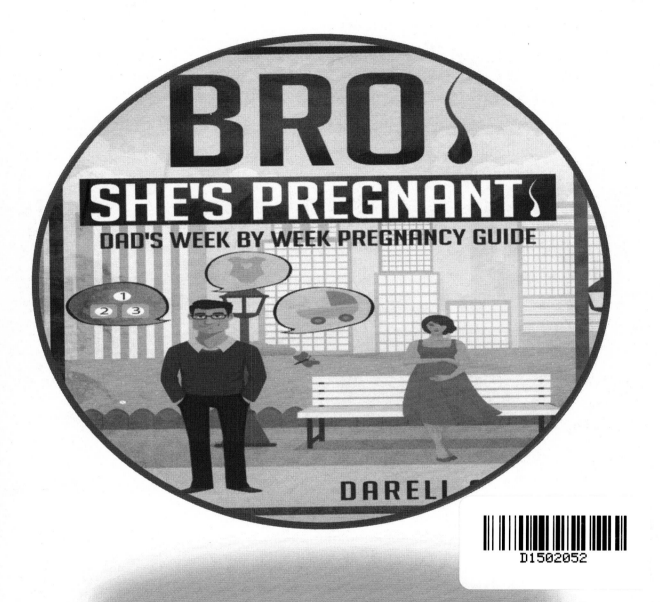

Contents

INTRODUCTION

Yipee……..your wife has announced that she is expecting!

Wow! Calls for a celebration, doesn't it?

You have been dreaming about this day for long and finally it has arrived!

Both you and your partner are on cloud nine. <u>But there's a little problem dude.</u>

While there are tons of resources and guide books available for your wife, you are struggling to understand things on your own. It's your first time and it has finally hit you that you are also expecting – although in a different manner. Your partner's pregnancy is bringing out emotions and feelings that you do not understand and there aren't too many resources that you could turn to.

It is important to understand that a man's emotional response to pregnancy is no less varied than a woman's. You actually feel everything – anger, joy, fear, frustration, relief, denial…

And to top this up, around eighty percent of men also experience physical symptoms of pregnancy.

Shocked? Well, we shall talk about this later in the book.

They say that the moment the pregnancy test stick turns blue, the light to fatherhood turns green. If this book is in your hand, chances are that you are either an expectant father or intentionally headed in that direction.

You and your partner are getting ready to hop in for a fast and furious bumpy ride that will be filled with chills, thrills, and of course numerous spills.

The primary objective of this book is to help you understand what you are going through so that you are better prepared and can stay involved throughout the pregnancy. Understanding your partner's perspective on pregnancy (and we are talking about physical and emotional perspective) is also essential to understand how you will react.

The information provided in this book is simple and straightforward. We shall divide each chapter into five parts:

Part one: What's happening with the baby?

This part of the book will provide you detailed information regarding your baby's growth and development – from the union of sperm and egg to a living, breathing infant.

Part two: What's happening with your partner?

But I thought the book was about me!

Sure, the book is about you. However, for you to stay involved throughout the pregnancy, it is critical to understand what your partner is going through and when.

Therefore, we shall begin each chapter summarizing your partner's physical and emotional experiences.

Part three: What's happening with you?

Well, that's what this book is about, isn't it? Pregnancy may impact your sex life and you may experience a number of changes – some good, others bad and yet others that you may feel indifferent to. Let's get a perspective.

Part four: How can you stay involved?

While part three covers the emotional and physical side of pregnancy, this one deals with specific tips that can help you make this pregnancy 'your own.' You will get to read some fascinating methods to communicate with the baby, have maximum fun and learning during the birthing classes and even learn some delicious and nutritious recipes to prepare

Part five: Preventing hunger pangs

Each month, you will get to learn five delicious recipes that you can prepare to ensure that your partner gets to relish the most delicious food on the planet even if she is not able to prepare it herself.

OKAY….BUT WHY SHOULD I GET INVOLVED?

The reason is simple – *Because it is good for your partner, your child and yourself!*

Research indicates that involvement during pregnancy is a great indicator of involvement after pregnancy.

Not only this, your involvement also helps your partner – your partner is more likely to breastfeed your baby if you are involved (and we all know why this is so important).

The bonus of getting involved is prevention from risky behavior. As a responsible would be dad, you begin to take better care of yourself, you are happier in your relationship and even outshine others at work.

You see yourself smoothly transition from a DUDE (someone who Didn't Understand Daunting Expectations) to a DAD (Determined And Dedicated).

CHAPTER TWO: THE FIRST TRIMESTER
WEEK 1 and 2: PRECONCEPTION FOR MEN

Parenting is a lot like marathon training. It is extremely exhausting and definitely a huge commitment. However, the reward that you experience once you cross that finish line cannot be described in words.

So, first things first – the moment you decide that you will begin the baby making process, you must begin to take care of yourself – think about your body like an athlete training for marathon.

The immediate step – head to your doctor for a check-up. Your partner does a number of things to get herself ready for this big step. You too need to think about this. Are you physically ready for this? How about varicose veins? Observe your body – do you notice any in the scrotum?

Varicose veins in the scrotum can alter your sperm count. You may even want to consider going easy on biking as it has been known to alter sperm counts. Using hot tubs may also become an issue.

You must check with your physician for advice on these specific topics.

A very important adjustment that you need to make is the mindset adjustment. You have to begin thinking not only about yourself but also about your family

Your partner may even ask you to make specific changes in your lifestyle. These may include incorporating healthier eating habits, quitting smoking and cutting off the junk from your food. You should also try and eliminate as many medicines as possible from your routine. The reason for this is that medicines such as Tegamet, Nitrofurantoin, etc. which are used to treat gastrointestinal disorders also impact the male fertility. Your sperm production and count may both be compromised. Yikes!

You may even be required to undergo genetic testing for conditions such as Down's syndrome, cystic fibrosis and Tay-Sachs and the 'actually I know it,' 'what if,' 'hopefully not,' etc. may play havoc on your mind for a few days (till the reports are out)

Think about how your partner patiently goes through tons of tests – there is so much that she endures – bodily changes, pain, anxiety, risks…the list is endless.

The least you can do here is help her through the process by arming yourself with information that may serve you for better.

And while you are doing all this prep, do not forget to do something that you really enjoy – you want to be physically fit and have a positive mindset too!

As you are trying to get pregnant, the last thing that your partner would like to hear is that you are not ready or cannot do it.

Remember, the fair amount of fear that both of you demonstrate is acceptable – but you only have nine months to get yourself ready – financially, emotionally and beyond.

Do not play the blame game if you do not succeed during the first few efforts. Think about how you achieved success when you had sex the first time – you were skeptical, it was terrifying but you rose to the challenge and did it, correct?

This is one of those times, you will have to rise to the challenge and use your sex drive and energy to stay on the top of your game.

Do not let the process of making babies become mechanical. Think about things that your partner likes doing, think about things that you can do to please her and make her feel great. Because, even though you are making babies, you are indirectly making love. Enjoy each other, eliminate the stress and have fun in each other's company.

A great tip here is to keep cool. Studies show that sperm counts increase by substantial amounts if you stop using the hot water tub. Wearing boxers instead of tight fitting shorts can also help here.

Steroids, heavy drinking, heavy tobacco smoking, heavy drinking and extreme emotional stress can all work together to decrease your sperm count. Try and eliminate these as much as possible.

Now, it is always advisable to keep realistic expectations when you are trying to get pregnant.

Well, she is wearing the sexiest lingerie and has put on an amazing lap dance for you as she refills your snifter and simultaneously encourages you to take off your boxers….that's such an awesome thought, isn't it?

Well, daddy-to-be, it is time to wake up! Your partner has decided to get pregnant and now there is nothing that can stop her. Therefore, your sexual preferences are not on the agenda for now.

Disheartened?

Don't be…she needs you at this time, she desires you…but she needs the baby too. And she is stressed out! She doesn't say so…but she is.

At this stage, understand that it is your partner who is actually getting pregnant. She must be under so much more pressure. Be like a rock for your partner, support her, be a great listener and allow her to vent out her problems at this time. Listen to her – she may have fears and she may have hopes. She may cry some day because she feels it's not happening and she may be extremely happy some other day, assuming that it is going to happen today.

Understanding how it all works:

Pretty much every month, your partner ovulates and her body is ready to have a baby. So, when your sperm gets to meet her egg, the party in her uterus begins.

The good news here is that as a couple intending to get pregnant, you get a clear window to behave like rabbits each month.

The bad news is that certain factors can reduce your chances of pregnancy and this may result in loads of frustration.

We have already looked at the factors that can impact your sperm count.

Here is a personal question:

Are you like most men, who when she offers an oral are like – *'Yeah baby….I wanna cum in your mouth!!!'*

Well, if that is the case, here is a revelation – Oral stimulation can reduce your chances of pregnancy since her saliva kills your soldiers (sperms).

She loves it when you put that weird lubricant on your stick!

Not any more…That thing can also reduce your chances of conception and conception is more important to her than anything else at this point in time, isn't it?

So, throw that bottle away while you are preparing to get pregnant.

So, what's the solution?

The only solution here is to have smart sex and not hard sex. The ovulation kit available at your local chemist will help your partner know that her egg is ready to launch.

Now is the time to get your soldiers into the battlefield.

Whether it is an early Sunday morning or a Thursday afternoon, when the kit asks you to have sex, you must comply.

Sounds hot, huh?

Well, strangely it is not as hot as it sounds. The process sometimes becomes so mechanical that you begin to feel used for sex.

But that's okay…talk to your partner, love her and reinforce your commitment to get pregnant.

When to seek medical assistance?

Well, you have been trying for a year and are still not pregnant? Now is the time to move over to the next step – seeking medical assistance.

Depending on why your sperm and her egg are not uniting, you doctor may prescribe certain medications. One such medication is Clomid. The side effect – your partner's hormone levels shoot up – you see that fire in her eyes and you plant your seed into her womb. If luck has it, you get pregnant.

If not, you move to the next step – a visit to an infertility specialist. This is a weird part – you may be asked to give blood for some tests, and then you may be given a cup along with some outdated adult materials. You are now supposed to fill this cup with your precious fluid.

I sincerely hope that you are able to work with Mother Nature and avoid all of this.

In a scenario where you do have to undergo this, the stress to achieve results goes up. And you are not the only one feeling this. Your partner probably takes the blame on herself and is ten times more stressed than you. Each failed attempt disheartens her and breaks her confidence.

This is the time for you to 'get in the zone.' Light some candles, sniff some chamomile and just be there for her – whenever she needs you.

WEEK 3 AND 4: YIPEE, I AM PREGNANT!
Wow…she suspects that she is pregnant.

Her next step - she sends you to the store to get the pregnancy test kit.

Remember, the pregnancy test game is an expensive game and women normally play it several times between the seven to twelve days of missing their period. You must set aside around $50 for this amazing game.

To prevent her from testing until the twelfth day may require immense effort – may be a cage, a rope or something else…Whatever you say or do may not impact and she may begin the process of testing on the seventh day itself. In fact, she may take several tests on day number seven – even if most of them come out as negative. Remember, the test can be negative on the seventh day even if she is really pregnant.

Another point of consideration is that even if the test comes out as positive, she may take several more tests – *just to be sure*.

For you, this means several trips to your local pharmacy.

If all goes well, at some point you will receive the good news – *Yay! She is pregnant.*

This is the time that you feel that unique emotion that bonds all first time fathers together. You feel like you have hit the million dollar jackpot. Your mind is colored with fear and little anxiousness too.

Secretly, you are relieved too! You have finally made it...you are even proud that you made your partner pregnant – this proves that you are a fully functional man, may be a stud as well.

In case you are not the biological father of your child and your partner conceived through Assisted Reproductive Techniques, you will feel a different kind of a relief. Those visits to infertility clinics, those ups and downs, those hopes and disappointments now seem to be a thing of past.

You indulge in self talk – *Will you be able to handle the challenge?*

Yeah...I will be fine, I am prepared.

Well, It's a big responsibility.

Yeah...but my work is over, no? Now it is the mom-to-be's job to ensure that things are smooth for the next nine months.

No, dude you are mistaken. You are now a Dad. And believe it or not – it does take effort to get your kid launched.

However, here is some good news – With love, hard work and a little help, you can venture into this brand new world without any problem.

WHAT'S HAPPENING WITH YOU - YOUR REACTION MATTERS!

She just told you that she is pregnant! You are on cloud nine. Do you want to shake a martini or open some wine?

Well, slow down Dad.

Sounds a little unfamiliar, correct?

Dad sounds unfamiliar and slowing down is not your thing.

Starting now, you will have to make changes in your thought process.

You must remember that your partner cannot drink alcohol. If you really need a drink, seek her permission to enjoy one. My suggestion is to refrain from drinking as a gesture of solidarity.

And now you are thinking – *God! I did not sign up for this. How long is this going to last?*

Well, traditionally that number is 40 weeks from the date of her last period. Your doctor will provide an official 'due date' based on the information she provides them.

Remember, the due date is not written in stone – it can change depending on a number of other factors.

Now that you realize that fatherhood is just around the corner, you may feel that unexplained pressure getting built up. This may even lead to unnecessary anxiety or fear.

Take a deep breath and look at first time dads around you. Notice how happy they feel when they are in the company of their little one – similar to them, you are going to love being a dad more than you think.

Think about how you would be about to leave for work and he will call you 'Daddy' for the very first time.

Think about how you would arrive home after attending a hectic business meeting and the smile on your child's face will simply make you forget about the 'not so good day at work.'

There will be numerous such moments – the joys are simply unlimited – let the process of visualization begin!

WHAT'S HAPPENING WITH HER – HER REACTION TOO!

Your partner may feel a hundred emotions at one time. You are extremely excited as you think – Wow, she is pregnant!

While she is thinking about the best way to nurture the child within her, labor pain, the changes in her body and the manner in which she would groom her child.

She is already thinking about the school your child would go to, the clothes they would wear at a particular event and so on…

She experiences a heightened feeling of closeness to you. You may also get to notice her sudden mood swings and there will be times when she will cry for no reason.

Physically, she may begin to experience some or all of the following symptoms:

- Morning sickness (vomiting, nausea and heartburn)
- Food aversions
- Food cravings
- Headaches, irritability, dizziness
- Breast changes (tenderness and enlargement)
- Fatigue

Almost ninety percent of women experience morning sickness and nausea, heartburn or vomiting catches them at any hour of the day.

Most women also experience that their morning sickness gets better after the first trimester. Here are a few things that you can do to help:

- Begin with the good news. Did you know that women who experience morning sickness are less likely to have low birth weight babies? The risks of miscarriage and premature labor are also minimized. Research also indicates that the babies IQ is directly proportional to the severity of symptoms.
- Encourage her to keep herself hydrated. Caffeine is naturally dehydrating. Therefore, encourage her to begin the day with some non-acidic fruit juice or flat soda.
- Help her maintain a nourishing high protein, high carbohydrate diet.
- Encourage her to consume loads of nutritious small meals in the day – may be four or five small meals. She should eat every three hours if possible. And always try and eat before she feels nauseated.
- Take her out for a walk. Some women feel relived with walking.
- Make sure that she is taking all her prenatal vitamins.
- Put some crackers, pretzels and rice cake near her bedside. She will need something to begin and end the day with.
- You may even want to look at alternative treatment options. Do not get involved in anything that is too risky.

HOW CAN YOU STAY INVOLVED?

Exercise:

Getting exercise during pregnancy is critical. It will improve your partner's blood circulation and keep her energy levels up.

Exercise has been known to contribute towards better sleep patterns, mood elevation and reduction of other pregnancy related discomforts. In case your partner was working out prior to getting pregnant, she will not need any encouragement to exercise. She must just continue to do what she was doing. However, if your partner has never worked out till now, pregnancy must not be an excuse to lie down on the sofa day in and day out. Tell her the benefits that she would experience and be a supportive partner – being with her as she exercises. Exercise improves strength and endurance which comes in handy during delivery.

Here are some fun ways to exercise together:

- Walking
- Running
- Low impact aerobics
- Swimming or water aerobics
- Cycling
- Tennis
- Light weight lifting
- Yoga (no extreme stretches please)

Do consult your practitioner before beginning to exercise and remember to keep yourself hydrated throughout.

Nutrition:

Did you read about the food pyramid in grade six? Well, the basics of nutrition still remain the same. Remember that your partner is pregnant and will need an extra 300 calories per day. If she is carrying multiples, she might need to eat even more – consult your doctor for advice.

In case she was overweight before getting pregnant, this is not the time to go on a diet. At the same time, this is also not an excuse to 'eat for two.'

The average woman requires around 45 gm. of protein per day. However, your pregnant partner may need around 80 gm. of protein. Nutritionists believe that a high protein diet during the first nineteen weeks of pregnancy supports the surge in brain cell growth in the baby. Lean protein and low fat milk is your best bet.

At least three servings of iron rich food are recommended. Legumes, fortified cereals, spinach and dried fruit are good sources of iron. Her prenatal vitamins could also contain an extra dose of iron. Encourage her to take these with some orange juice which will facilitate the process of absorption.

At least seven servings of fruits and vegetables are recommended.

Calcium is critical for your baby's bones. Since a major a part of your partner's calcium intake goes directly to the baby, she needs to get enough for herself. Milk, pink salmon, tofu, broccoli and calcium fortified orange juice constitute some great options.

Green and yellow vegetables are extremely important and will help your partner absorb all the extra protein that she will be eating. The darker the green, the better it is for her.

Grains are fuel for her body and at least four servings are required during the day. If she won't have enough fuel, there may not be enough for the baby. The high fiber content in grains can prevent her from constipation. Great sources of grains include brown rice, whole grain breads, quinoa, dried beans, peas and potatoes.

At least eight or more glasses of water are recommended for consumption every day.

You partner must consume some fat too. Monounsaturated fats such as avocado, canola oil, olive oil and peanuts are good for her. However, not more than 30 percent of her total caloric intake should come from fat.

Definite no's:

Alright, here is the deal – if your partner eats something, drinks something or smells something, so does your growing baby.

When a mom-to-be inhales cigarettes, her womb fills with nicotine, tar, carbon monooxide and resins that inhibit oxygen and nutrient delivery to the baby. This enhances the risk of low birth weight babies and miscarriages.

And now, don't think that you can continue to smoke. Paternal smoking is equally bad and impacts your baby in a negative manner.

Bottom line – *if you are a smoker, now is the time to quit*. If your partner is a smoker, encourage her to quit and help her however you can.

When it comes to alcohol, complete abstinence is the safest choice. Some practitioners do sanction an occasional glass of wine to induce relaxation. Regular, high dose of alcohol consumption can lead to fetal alcohol syndrome and your baby may be born with certain irreversible physical and mental impairments and abnormalities.

Your partner must never go on a 24 hour fast. The reason for this is the rapid development in your baby's brain cells during the first nineteen weeks of pregnancy.

She should consult her doctor prior to taking any over the counter medicine such as aspirin, ibuprofen or the regular cold medicines.

It is extremely important to avoid caffeine during the first few months of pregnancy. Caffeine not only dehydrates you, but also elevates the risk of miscarriage or premature birth.

You and your partner must not consume any recreational drugs during pregnancy. Remember, your unborn child may be born addicted!

Your partner must avoid raw meat, fish or eggs. She should not consume unpasteurized milk throughout her pregnancy.

Helping your partner eat a highly nutritious diet is the best thing you can do to ensure that you have a healthy and happy baby. Also remember, that she will be better off eating nothing but healthy foods all the time, an occasional order of fries or candy bar will not lead to a long term damage. So, be supportive in whatever way you can be.

If you are one of those fathers who has used assisted reproductive techniques for child birth and get to meet the surrogate, encourage her to make healthy lifestyle and nutritional choices.

FIGHTING THOSE HUNGER PANGS

You will be amazed at how quickly your partner would begin to feel hungry. Even if she has had an evening snack, she could demand for something else before dinner.

Now, if you have been doing most of the cooking in your house, things won't change much. But, if she has been involved with the cooking, then you need to make some changes in order to make life comfortable for her. You must learn to cook simple, quick and nutritious meals. You may have to go shopping for ingredients as you do the meal planning. Even if your partner still takes care of the cooking, ensure that your help her with shopping for ingredients. Try and make her a nutritious breakfast shake. She might need those extra ten minutes of relaxation in bed. Some granola bars, candies and dried fruit in the glove compartment will come out really handy when you have to travel together.

Let us look at some quick recipes that you can make to ensure that she is satiated all the time:

Recipe 1: Breakfast shake: Combine 1 banana, 10 strawberries, juice of 1 orange and ¾ cup skim milk in a blender or a food processer. Serve chilled over ice.

Recipe 2: Peel and slice carrots and keep them in a transparent box in the refrigerator. She can snack whenever she wants to and they are visible.

Recipe 3: Nutritious egg salad: Half three hard boiled eggs and mix with dried fruit, sunflower seeds, nuts and raisins. Season with Himalayan salt, oregano and paprika.

Recipe 4: Quinoa cherry porridge: Take a medium sized pan and stir together ½ cup quinoa, ½ cup dried cherries, a pinch of cinnamon and 1 cup water. Bring this mixture to boil over a medium-high flame. Reduce the heat to simmer and continue to cook for approximately fifteen minutes until all water is absorbed and quinoa is tender. Drizzle with a tablespoon of honey and serve with some natural ginger tea!

Recipe 5: Breakfast blueberry omelet: To start with, microwave 2 slices of turkey bacon as per the instructions provided on the packet. Now, mix ½ cup beaten egg whites, ¼ cup low fat Ricotta cheese, a pinch of cinnamon, 1 tablespoon of silvered almonds, ½ cup blueberries and 2 teaspoons of vanilla extract in a bowl. Next, pour into a heated skillet that has been sprayed with some cooking oil. Cook like an omelet and pour ½ cup blueberries as toppings over the omelette. Enjoy!

WEEK 5 TO 8: HONEY, WE NEED TO SEE A DOCTOR!

Alright so finally the feeling of fatherhood is sinking in. Life is not too difficult, it's just the mood swings and her morning sickness and her breasts…oh…her breasts look enlarged…but the sex drive seems to be fading away…on some days okay..

WHAT'S HAPPENING WITH THE BABY?

During this month, the baby changes from an embryo into a fetus. They will have a tiny little heart, stubby little arms (without any fingers) with wrists closed and sealed shut eyes on the side of the face.

WHAT'S HAPPENING WITH HER?

Well, she is getting apprehensive now. She knows her size will increase and has a strange fear – fear that you won't love her anymore. She is unable to concentrate on her work and demonstrates mixed feelings – feelings or elation as well as of fear. She has a strange fear of miscarriage and her mood swings continue during this month too.

Physically, she demonstrates the below mentioned symptoms:

- Continued morning sickness
- Continued fatigue
- Tingling in fingers
- Tenderness around breasts
- Enlargement of breasts
- Darkening of nipples
- Frequent urination

AND WHAT'S HAPPENING WITH YOU?

Well, women 'connect' with their pregnancies sooner than men do. The pregnancy seems to be more 'real' for them. They don't experience the baby kicking but their bodies undergo physical changes which makes them believe something is happening. For most men, pregnancy at month two is an abstract thing – in fact, so abstract that they may even forget it at times. Once it sinks in, you experience mixed feelings – you may be really elated at times – in fact, you may want to stop strangers and tell them that you are going to be a father. You visualize playing catch with your child, taking them out for a bike ride, teaching them how to swim…the list goes on and on.

On the other hand you are secretly scared of miscarriage and therefore do not want to get attached to the idea so soon.

Pregnancy and sex

Well, you will notice a change in your sex life – and it will be a drastic change. Some men look at pregnancy as a reconfirmation of their masculinity and as a result experience an increased sexual desire. It also stems from the fact that they do not have to now worry about birth control. This can lead to increased passion and love, resulting in wilder sex during the earlier months of pregnancy.

However, all men do not experience similar symptoms. Some are turned off by their partners changing figure whereas the others may be worried about hurting the baby or their partner.

Whatever you are experiencing with respect to sex, talk about it with your partner. It is quite likely that she is also experiencing or will shortly experience something similar.

Some men also start getting wilder dreams – they dream of wild sex with their partner, ex-girlfriend or even a prostitute. This is because you are concerned that your partner's pregnancy may hamper your sex life, or may be even enhance it. Do not discuss your dreams with your partner.

Your partner may also sometimes experience a strange heightened sex drive – so be ready for that commercial break in 'The Big Bang Theory' to convert into a 'between the sheets' event for you and your partner.

HOW CAN YOU STAY INVOLVED?

The general rule that women connect with their babies sooner than men has one exception – *men who get involved during the early stages of pregnancy and stay involved until the end, connect with their babies better.* One way to stay involved is by accompanying your partner for each doctor visit. It is an awesome opportunity to get answers to your questions and also understand the things that are going inside your partner's womb.

These visits to the doctor will generate greater involvement and over a course of time, you will being to view this pregnancy as your 'own.' It also tends to demystify the whole process. At month three, you will be able to hear your baby's heartbeat for the first time – the feeling that you will experience at this time cannot be described in words.

If you are one of those unfortunate couples who have had to experience a previous miscarriage, you may see yourself getting unnecessarily tensed about how things will go this time. Try not to worry. Only one in two hundred couples experience miscarriage repeatedly and you are not going to be that one. Do not pay attention to other people's horror stories and don't spill the beans until you are ready to. Only tell your friends and family when you feel completely ready to talk about your pregnancy. Ask your doctor for additional ultrasounds to listen to your baby's heart beat – it is definitely reassuring. Get some support and support your partner too. Try to keep her calm and stay calm too.

Oh....the mandatory tests!

Over a period of time, your partner will expect you to be there for her always. While a visit to a doctor may not sound like a romantic idea, it reassures her that you care and that you love her.

Since you will be accompanying your partner in all her check-ups, creating a schedule helps.

You must know that if all goes well, you would have to visit the doctor every month for the first six months and every other week during month seven and eight. Post month eight, you will need the visit the doctor every week until she delivers.

In case you are not able to take time off from work on these days, check with the doctor on early morning or late evening appointments.

Your partner will have to take a number of tests during these nine months – the scariest of these are the tests to diagnose any birth defects. Your doctor will take a thorough history and based on what you tell them, they might order some extra prenatal tests (that is if you are in the high risk category).

The ultra sonogram is a non-invasive test that can be performed any time after week five. It lets you see the picture of your baby along with the placenta. The 2-D images may seem vague to the untrained eye. The 3-D ones are a little clearer where you can see the complete picture of your fetus. The 4-D images allow you to see your future baby in action – sucking his thumb or trying to swim.

An ultrasound is normally not recommended in the first trimester except when your doctor suspects something that is out of the blue.

At this stage you get a confirmation on the presence of pregnancy.

The second trimester ultrasounds are more reliable. Some couples get these done to know the sex of the baby (this is an optional thing). These ultrasounds also provide an idea of the due date.

Additional ultrasounds are ordered during the third trimester to get an idea on the positon of the baby or the amount of amniotic fluid that supports the baby.

Now, you are not pregnant. But you may have to get yourself pricked by the needle a number of times. Certain blood tests are performed on both parents to ensure that there are no genetic defects in your 'to be born' child. Certain ethnic groups are more susceptible to certain genetic diseases than the others. Sickle cell anemia, Thalassemia, Cystic fibrosis and Canavan disease can easily be diagnosed through prenatal testing of both partners.

You would also need to be tested if your partner's blood group is Rh-ve and your blood group is Rh+ve.

Amniocentesis is a test performed at 15-18 weeks and can diagnose every possible chromosomal abnormality. I would suggest getting this done at a lab that does maximum number of procedures. Another test called CVS can be performed a lot earlier than amniocentesis and helps you identify any potential chromosomal abnormalities. It also gives the 'parents to be' more time to think about options.

And what if...

Well, around 1-2 percent of the embryos that do not embed in the uterus find a place outside the womb and settle there. (The pregnancy is termed as an *ectopic pregnancy* in this case). Usually, the secure place is the fallopian tube where they try to attach and grow. Since the Fallopian tube is unable to accommodate the growing size of the fetus, it may just burst leading to severe bleeding. Fortunately, most ectopic pregnancies are caught and removed by the eighth week – much before they become dangerous.

And wait...before you get your thinking hats on...there is absolutely no way to transplant this embryo into the uterus. Therefore, the only option that you are left with is to terminate the pregnancy.

Your partner may also experience protein induced hypertension or *preeclampsia*. Women with history of high blood pressure are prone to preeclampsia. Headache, water retention, blurred vision, pain in abdomen and seizures are some of the symptoms that your woman may get if she experiences preeclampsia.

Unfortunately there is no guaranteed way to prevent this but ensuring that she monitors her salt intake, stays well hydrated and gets enough exercise can help her.

How about birth defects?

If as a result of testing, you get an indication about a possible deformity in your baby, you and your partner have two options ahead of you: you can either terminate the pregnancy or keep the baby. You may need the help of genetic counselors in order to make this decision.

Don't be afraid to seek professional support in order to help yourself and your partner deal with grief. Going to a support group can help too.

FIGHTING HUNGER PANGS IN MONTH TWO

Well, a big part of staying involved is to stay involved with her exercise, hydration and nutritional needs. Here are some more recipes that you may want to experiment with:

Recipe 1: Orange and apple breakfast juice: Blend together 2 oranges (peeled and deseeded), 1 apple (peeled and cored), 1 inch ginger root, ½ beetroot and 1 tablespoon flax seed. Pour in a tall glass and enjoy. This healthy breakfast option is full of omega 3 fatty acids and also contains the fiber from flax which helps in fighting constipation.

Recipe 2: Easy peasy pumpkin soup: Place the crockpot over medium high heat and pour in ½ a cup of vegetable broth, ½ cup chopped onion, 2 cloves minced garlic and 1 inch minced ginger root. Bring this to boil and then cook on simmer for five minutes. Pour in 2 cups of pumpkin puree, 1 ½ cup of vegetable stock, ½ teaspoon fresh thyme and 1 teaspoon salt. Cook for around thirty minutes. Puree the soup using a handheld blender. Remove from heat, garnish with ½ teaspoon fresh parsley and serve with some green salad.

Recipe 3: Roasted veggies: You will need 2 cups butternut squash (peeled and deseeded), 1 cup Yukon gold potato (unpeeled and cubed), 1 cup beetroot (unpeeled and cubed), 1 cup broccoli (cut into half inch pieces), 1 medium sized red onion (chopped), around 7 garlic cloves (minced) and two tablespoon olive oil. Preheat the oven to 425 degrees. Take two baking sheets and oil them with olive oil. Combine all the above mentioned ingredients in a large salad bowl and toss them. Spread these over the prepared baking sheets and sprinkle pepper and salt. Roast the veggies for around one hour. You may serve immediately or store in a casserole for a day, re-warm it for fifteen minutes and serve the next day!

Recipe 4: Flax and Dill sauce: A great source of protein and omega 3 fatty acids, this sauce makes a perfect dip for her crackers and veggies. You would need 1/3 cups of low fat yogurt, ½ teaspoon olive oil, ½ tablespoon ground flaxseed, 1 teaspoon minced garlic and 1 teaspoon Dill. Simply combine these ingredients together in a blender and enjoy with sliced carrots and apples.

Recipe 5: Strawberry freezer pops: She might just get a craving for something sweet. Surprise her with these super easy freezer pops. Take 2 tablespoons crushed almonds and around 15 strawberries and blend well in a food processor. Add three cups of plain low fat yogurt and blend again. Pour into six paper cups and insert a popsicle stick into each cup. Freeze overnight. Before eating, just tear the paper cup. Isn't it mouth-watering?

WEEK 9 TO 12: SPILLING THE BEANS – YUP! THE PREGNANCY IS 'REAL'!

This is the month when you will want to actually let your friends and family know about your partner's pregnancy. (In fact, a good number of dad's to be begin talking about it as 'their own' pregnancy by this month).

WHAT'S HAPPENING WITH THE BABY?

By now, your little fetus has started looking like a real person, except for the fact that it is only around two to three inches long and weighs less than an ounce. The fetus has a gigantic head (now, gigantic is a relative term – in reality, the head is only the size of a grape). The internal organs are developing too. By the end of this month, your baby will be able to curl their toes, turn their heads and breathe amniotic fluid.

WHAT'S HAPPENING WITH HER?

She has heard the baby's heartbeat. Now, there is a heightened sense of reality. She is still experiencing mood swings and sometimes gets worried on how she would get through the remaining six months. She is also concerned about her increasing waistline and wonders if she will ever return to her original figure. She has begun to bond with the baby and even talks to them. She is concerned about the things happening inside her stomach and is trying to gain as much information as possible. All she cares about now is the baby and their safety.

Physically, her breast continue to enlarge and remain tender. She continues to experience morning sickness, nausea and fatigue. She does not appear to be pregnant but has trouble fitting in her clothes.

WHAT'S HAPPENING WITH YOU?

By this time, you begin to view your partner's pregnancy as your own. The heart beat that you heard at the doctor's clinic helps in making you believe that the pregnancy actually exists.

You may even have your moments of doubt – when you are not too excited about the whole thing. At times, you may be worried if all is going to be alright with your partner and the baby. Questions such as 'Will I be able to make it on time?' are playing havoc on your mind.

Until now, you have been the center of your partner's universe. Now, you may get worried that the entire focus might shift to the baby. You may even fear losing your independence, sex life or savings.

Do not be surprised if you begin to develop physical symptoms of pregnancy. You would be surprised to know that around 90 percent of American fathers experience physical symptoms of pregnancy. This is referred to as the *couvade syndrome* and the symptoms are traditionally similar to those of a pregnant woman – weight gain, headache, diarrhea, cysts, mood swings, and even hunger pangs. Usually, these symptoms appear for the first time during the third month of pregnancy and then disappear during the second trimester, only to come back again in the third trimester. It's a mystery how these symptoms disappear at birth.

One of the reasons why you are experiencing these symptoms is because you want to take your partner's pain away. You are really stressed out about the discomfort that she may be experiencing and sometimes feel that you are responsible for her being in such a miserable condition.

Some men are used to all the attention in the relationship and cannot cope up with attention shifting towards their lady during the process of childbirth. In this case, these symptoms may just appear as a result of this unexplained, unwanted and unintentional jealousy.

Some men are even susceptible to hormone changes.

But you thought that it was only your partner who would get impacted this way!

True! Although the impact of hormones is much more pronounced in your partner, you may also experience your prolactin and cortisol level rise up.

Did you know that through these symptoms you could be secretly telling your partner that you are there for her? A number of women worry if their partner is going to be there for them.

While you can stay involved by talking to her, accompanying her on her prenatal visits, cleaning the house for her, cooking for her and generally pampering her, if you are overly stressed, these symptoms could be your way of showing her how involved you are.

Now, I am not saying that you should get these symptoms. However, this could be one of the reasons why you get them.

HOW CAN YOU STAY INVOLVED?

Most people inform their friends and family about their pregnancy during this month. Make sure that 'my wife is pregnant' status that you typed on Facebook becomes 'we are expecting' before you press the 'post' button. This is one way of letting your partner know that you are in this with her.

Be prepared for unexpected guests at home, who would just stop by to see how things are progressing and of course the phone will ring more than the usual. Most people will check on your partner's health and emotions and you may suddenly feel left out.

Well, you have three options here:

- *Option one*: Just sulk…and get some more attention ☺
- *Option two*: Just ignore…it's alright baby!
- *Option three*: (which is what I recommend) Become proactive and start talking to your guests on how excited you are and how you are also experiencing certain symptoms. Seek advice, be participative in all discussions and show your partner how she means the world to you.

Do not feel left out if your partner is spending loads of time talking about her pregnancy with her girlfriends and family. It is totally up to you to not let that happen. Try remaining the best friend you were by talking about the baby (a lot) with her.

Let your ob/gyne know that you want to stay involved and ask questions when you visit them every month. Do not miss her appointments. In fact, make them your own appointments.

Despite all the good things and the bonding that is happening between you and your partner, pregnancy is also a time of stress and can sometimes impact your relationship in a negative way.

Remember, she is experiencing changes in her body. She has had to give up on a number of things that she was used to (may be alcohol or smoking). Support her as much as you can and don't impose anything on her. Those weekly visits to the bar can definitely be curbed for nine months. All she needs is your support!

Time alone please: At this stage, you may be already bored with too many baby conversations. Almost everything in your house and friends circle seems to revolve around the baby. If this is the case, getting some time alone won't hurt at all. Before you head out of the house for your much needed break, make sure that your partner is aware of where you are going. You can decide to catch up with some old, childless friends or may be watch a play, or may be read something.

Always remember, that your partner is the one carrying your child. She may also need some time away from pregnancy. Make it up to her by preparing a sumptuous brunch or getting a thoughtful gift.

FIGHTING HUNGER PANGS IN MONTH THREE

Well, you will have to prepare some quick nutritional meals that satisfy your and your lady's taste buds. Here are your recipes for month three:

Recipe 1: Morning energy chocolate smoothie: You can begin by soaking 100gm. raw almonds and 25 gm cashews overnight. Begin the process of blending by blending together 2 handful of spinach, 1 ripe avocado, 200gm. coconut milk and 100 gm. almond milk. It should give you a smooth paste. Next, blend in the almonds, cashews and 1 tablespoon sunflower seeds. Now, add 2 tablespoons yogurt, 1 tablespoon cacao and 1 tablespoon maca powder. Maca powder has a strong taste, so experiment with a little amount first. You may choose to eliminate this if you wish. Lastly, blend in 3 tablespoons of coconut oil. Your ready to drink super energizing smoothie is ready in a jiffy! Enjoy!

Recipe 2: Grapefruit smoothie: You will need 2 grapefruits (peeled and deseeded), 1 cucumber (peeled and chopped), 1 avocado, 2 cups baby spinach (torn), 4 ounces of water and a pinch of stevia. Blend these together in a food processor or high speed blender to create your power packed smoothie.

Recipe 3: Mint and watercress lunch salad: You would need 100gm watercress, 100gm. rocket, 100gm. chickpeas (boiled or canned), ½ bunch fresh mint, 2 tablespoons each of olive oil and fresh lemon juice, Himalayan salt and pepper (to taste). Frist wash the leaves and dry over a kitchen tissue. Next arrange them in a salad serving and throw in the chickpeas over them. Complete by adding salt, pepper, lemon dressing and olive oil over the salad. Relish!

Recipe 4: Green dip for her crackers and veggies: This is the simplest dip or dressing that can be prepared. You would need 3 avocadoes, juice of 2 lemons, a handful each of Parsley and mint, 1 ½ cup spinach, ½ cup Pumpkin seeds, ¼ cup flax seeds, Himalayan salt and pepper to taste. Just put everything together in a blender and blend until smooth. Your delicious dip full of chlorophyll and alkaline minerals is ready to be enjoyed!

Recipe 5: Vegetable combo alkalizing lunch: You would need 4 carrots (peeled and cubed), 1 cup chopped fresh green beans, 1 cup fresh mushrooms, 1 teaspoon salt, ½ teaspoon thyme, 2 cloves of garlic and 2 tablespoons of raw non refined butter. Finely chop the garlic and stir fry in coconut oil or butter. Add the beans, mushrooms and carrot to the garlic and cook for approximately ten minutes, stirring continuously. Add the salt and thyme. Enjoy with any soup of your taste.

CHAPTER THREE: THE SECOND TRIMESTER

WEEK 13 TO WEEK 16: I CAN ONLY THINK ABOUT MONEY, HONEY!

By the time the fourth month kicks in, expectant dads begin to realize that they are 'actually' pregnant. The idea of pregnancy is now sinking in. If all goes well, this is the first time you will get to see your baby's ultrasound and watching that tiny heart pump will change everything for you.

WHAT'S HAPPENING WITH THE BABY?

During this month, the baby will grow to about four to five inches long and tip the scales at around 4 ounces. Their heart will pound away approximately 120-160 beats per minute and their whole body will be covered with small, smooth hair called *lanugo*. The fetus can swallow, kick or suck his thumb. Ultrasonic examinations reveal that they swallow their thumb when your partner eats sour food and suck it when they consume something sweet. They also begin to respond to light or dark.

WHAT'S HAPPENING WITH HER?

Well, she is extremely excited as she sees her sonogram and her worries about miscarriage begin to fade. Her mood swings continue and she appears forgetful at times. The responsibility of motherhood is slowly seeping in and she is anxious if she will be able to handle it. Something that seems like a good idea at 10:00am is a not so good idea at 10:15am. She needs you more than ever now. She wants reassurance that you will be there for her, always. She is concerned when her clothes don't fit her and seems to be obsessed with her figure.

Physically, her nipples will darken and so will any freckles and moles on her body. Her morning sickness will begin to settle down and you will notice her appetite returning – *for food as well as sex*! She may begin to experience heartburn which will be frequently triggered by eating. You may have to make certain changes on the food menu.

She may even become a little clumsy and drop and spill things and her vision may get impacted. Her contacts may bother her now and she may even get swelling in her gums (gingivitis). She may begin to feel light movements (but will not be able to make out that these are the baby movements). She may even begin to show – your friends will be able to now notice that tiny bump!

She may snore at times during the night and you may feel like going into a different room. That is definitely not a great idea. Always keep in mind that you signed up for this position of Daddy which demands at least two years of sleep deprivation.

At other times, she may just have difficulty in sleeping and will expect you to comfort her. Try getting her into an exercise program which can calm insomnia.

WHAT'S HAPPENING WITH YOU?

Well, you have now seen the ultrasound and the pregnancy seems to be real. Obviously, the significance of this pregnancy increases now!

At this time, you may even begin to feel that you are not yet ready for the baby. This feeling is common amongst expectant fathers who are in their early thirties or late twenties. They begin to worry about financial savings and how they would be able to provide for the child. Fathers over thirty five are mostly stable in their careers and therefore less bothered about this.

You may begin to work overtime and become obsessed by your job.

And if all this is not enough, your brain may be preoccupied with safety concerns – you are concerned if your partner and baby are doing fine, you are concerned if they are getting enough rest and if they are regular for their work outs. You may even start checking your partner's sleeping position.

My advice here would be to relax – slow down, dad – she is doing just fine! She understands that she needs to take care of herself and wants you to be there. But constant nagging is something that she does not appreciate.

Here are some ideas that can reassure her that you love her loads and make her the envy of her friends and family. Don't forget to continue using some of these even when she has delivered your baby. She deserves it!

- Nod and smile in agreement when she tells you that you do not have an idea of what it feels to be pregnant. She is right there!
- Write a letter to your unborn baby.
- Buy her an interesting name book.
- Keep reminding her that she is beautiful and do that every single day.
- Pay extra attention to her nutritional needs – pack some snacks for her before you both head out for shopping or other things.
- Learn some easy recipes and prepare at least one meal every day.
- Sign the two of you up for a childbirth preparation class.
- Do something with her that she knows you hate doing.
- Journal your thoughts about this pregnancy.
- Buy her a Mother's day or a Valentine's day gift – so what if it's only August!
- Never miss a prenatal appointment.
- Pick up her type of a movie, make some popcorn and curl up to watch it together – force yourself even if it is not your type.
- Stop smoking.
- Offer her a foot massage or a back rub.
- Get her manicure and pedicure appointments booked and go along with her, if possible.

- Don't let her see the unnecessary laundry around the house. Do it before it piles up, then fold it and keep it away.
- Hand over the TV remote to her and watch what she wants to watch.
- If she arrives home after you, have a candlelight dinner on the table.
- Frame the first ultrasound pic of the baby.
- Thank her for making you the happiest man on earth.
- Wipe her tears if she has an unexpected meltdown.
- Indulge her cravings.
- Leave some love notes around the house.
- Organize a surprise baby shower for her.
- Buy a pretty baby dress, gift wrap it and let her unwrap it. You will love the joy in her eyes.
- Remind her every day that she is going to be a great mother.
- Hold her hand while you are out walking.
- Put together a list of local take away restaurants.
- Plan a baby naming ceremony.
- Plan a romantic, weekend getaway. This would be the last time for quite a while.
- Write her a love letter and send it to her in mail.
- Kiss her – every day – long, sensual kisses…
- Give her loads of hugs.
- Gift her a spa treatment.
- Get her roses for no reason.
- Get her the most moisturizing bubble bath you can find.
- Buy her a maternity pillow.
- Go shopping with her for cute little maternity outfits and admire her as she wears them.
- Offer to pick up pizza on your way home from work and surprise her with her favorite ice cream too.
- Let her win all the arguments.
- Take a day off from work and just hang around the house with her.
- Surprise her with power shakes every other day.
- Treat her to a nice Sunday breakfast in bed.
- Never tell her that she looks tired (even if she does). In fact, offer to sleep early or get cozy with her in the bed.
- Let her know that she is sexy. Remind her every other day.
- Chocolates, flowers, jewelry…whatever your budget allows, just get them for her.
- Paint the baby's room and help her organize the crib.
- Listen to all her complaints but never tell her that she is complaining.
- Make a new will that includes your baby.
- Clean the closets and make space for baby clothes.
- Stay away from nasty comments like – *But you just had food?* Or *You look fat!* Remember, _it's not fat! It's not fat! And it's not fat! – that is the rule!_

HOW CAN YOU STAY INVOLVED?

Well, the very first rule of staying involved is to 'focus on her and her needs' at the moment. Remember, she needs you – she needs you to tell her that she is beautiful, that she is a great partner and that she will be the most awesome mother. Demonstrate your love to her in as many ways as you can. Demonstrate sensitiveness towards her changing physical appearance and emotions. Reassure her that she will lose all the baby fat and look even sexier once she delivers the baby. Tell her that she looks cute and sexy with the baby bump.

You must also discuss funding for your child's college education with your partner. You may want to start keeping aside some money every month so that your child does not have to struggle as they begin college. My suggestion here is to keep some money aside in your retirement account. This will reduce the liability on your child as they begin education and look at financial support options. You may also be able to withdraw money from your IRA in order to support their college education.

But before you begin the process of planning a retirement fund, you must take care of your present debts. Try paying them off as early as possible in order to secure your present.

You may even think about getting help from a professional financial counselor who can guide you how best to make financial decisions.

This is also a good time for you to reevaluate your life insurance cover. Remember, you are the provider and you need to ensure that your family members are taken care of in case of a mishap. And it is not too early to do that.

You may have to look at your will too. A will is a document that spells out how you would like to divide your assets if you die. In most cases, it goes to your partner and God forbid, if something happens to her, it goes to your child. In this scenario, you may need to appoint a guardian to look after the child's interest. A number of parents tend to ignore these little things, leaving much to chance. Do not fall into that trap and secure your child's future today.

ADDRESSING HUNGER PANGS IN MONTH FOUR

Here are a few new recipes that you could try this month to induce variety into her meals:

Recipe 1: Kiwi and kale smoothie: Blend 2 kiwi, ½ orange, ½ frozen banana, 1 bunch kale, 2 raw eggs and ½ cup of water in a high speed blender. Enjoy in a tall glass!

Recipe 2: Grilled salmon with chives, orange and black olives: You would need 4 center cut salmon fillet steaks, 1 tbsp. coconut oil, ½ tsp. sea salt, ½ tsp. ground pepper, ½ cup black olives, 2 oranges, ¼ cup chives, ½ fennel, 1 tbsp. olive oil and 1 lemon. Season the salmon fillet in pepper and sea salt. Grill on both sides using coconut oil. Keep for two minutes each side. Mix with other ingredients and dress with juice of 1 lemon and 1 tbsp. olive oil.

Recipe 3: Peppery salmons: You would need 4 skinless salmon fillets, 1 tbsp. lemon zest, 4 minced garlic cloves, 1 tbsp. extra virgin olive oil, 1 tsp. black pepper and 1 tsp. salt. Brush the salmon fillets on both sides with olive oil. Add the lemon zest over the salmon. Next, add the salt, pepper and garlic. Now, place this in a medium heated grill for eight minutes on each side. Serve with steamed broccoli, green salad, apples or avocados.

Recipe 4: Strawberry pancakes: Mash the two ripe bananas. Mix one egg into the batter. Whisk well and stir in the 1 tbsp. almond butter. Take a medium sized pan and pour one tbsp. coconut oil into it. Add a spoon full of pancake batter and cook over medium heat for four minutes on each side. Top with strawberries and relish your sumptuous breakfast.

Recipe 5: Mango dressing: Mix ½ cup extra virgin olive oil, ½ cup apple cider vinegar, ½ cup fresh mango, ½ tsp. paprika, ½ tsp. cayenne pepper and ¼ tsp. chili flakes. Blend well in a high speed blender and enjoy with crackers or fruits of choice.

WEEK 17 TO WEEK 20: CAN YOU HEAR ME, BABY?

This month, you may experience your baby's first gentle kick.

Yes! *That's the amazing reality*…you definitely are going to be a father and your child has begun their movements. Wow – *What an incredible feeling that it is!*

WHAT'S HAPPENING WITH THE BABY?

The baby still cannot open their eyes. However, their eyebrows and eyelashes are fully grown now. You may even be able to see some hair on their head. They experience occasional bouts of hiccups and are approximately nine inches long by the end of month five. They weigh around a pound and have now begun to grab the umbilical cord, kick or punch the mother's uterus. They sleep for around 95% of the time. Most of the awake time is spent in practicing somersaults.

WHAT'S HAPPENING WITH HER?

Well, she is experiencing baby movements 24/7 now and feels reassured about her pregnancy. There is absolutely no fear of miscarriage and she is overwhelmed with the advice that she is getting from almost everybody. She loves the attention that she receives in local trains, buses and grocery stores as people get up to give her a seat or help her with the bags. The baby bump increases and although she loves those feelings of motherhood, she is increasingly worried about her changing figure. Will she ever be able to look non pregnant?

She spends a lot of time daydreaming about the baby and develops a special bond with them – she wants to talk about each movement that she experiences.

She needs you to be there for her. Her sexual drive increases and she experiences less tenderness in her breasts now, although they continue to enlarge. Her breasts may also leak as she experiences a sexual urge. She is increasingly dependent on you – emotionally and physically – she needs a lot of support.

Physically, she may also experience occasional painless tightening of the uterus. These are called **Braxton Hicks contractions** or **false labor**. These do not follow a regular timing and are generally eased by change in position or walking.

Her nipples continue to darken and a dark line may appear down her belly button to the abdomen.

The fluid retention may change the shape of her eyeballs and her contacts may no longer fit her.

Hormones are causing other problems too – she is experiencing brittleness in her fingernails and has become increasingly forgetful.

But her hair looks amazing! In fact, they have never looked so great!

WHAT'S HAPPENING WITH YOU?

Alright, so you are finally going to be a father! Excitement will kick in once again as your partner places your hand on her belly and you experience a gentle kick.

As this initial excitement fades away, you begin to worry once again. You are worried if your baby is alright, if they are protected, if they are developed fully and if they are receiving the nutrition that they should be receiving!

Relax…Let me talk a little bit about the five senses that your baby will be born with and how they are working with their mother to ensure that they are perfect when they come out to see the world.

The sense of touch: Skin is considered as the body's largest organ. Your baby's skin is formed around two months into the pregnancy. Sensitivity begins with cheeks and lips and the baby turns towards the touch, whenever they are touched. This is referred to as the *rooting reflex* in infants and is used to find the breasts. When touched on the mouth, the baby begins working with nipples but also uses their hands to hold the breast. Fetuses spend a lot of time exploring themselves in order to develop their sense of touch. They hold the umbilical cord, suck on their fingers, stroke their face and kick against the walls of the uterus.

The sense of smell and taste: Once the baby's mouth and tongue developed (which is a few months ago), their taste buds are just as sensitive as yours. For the last few months, your baby has been drinking some amniotic fluid every day – they gulp in down their throat and then throw it out. After some time they drink this amniotic fluid once again. Don't start imagining it…..it may not be the most beautiful sight!

The taste and nasal flavors of the amniotic fluid change depending on what your partner eats. As the baby comes out of the womb, their sense of smell enables them to adjust to the life outside. Mommy's nipples smell like amniotic fluid and this is what attracts them to her breasts.

__The sense of hearing__: Believe it or not, the uterus is a pretty noisy place and it has been like that through the beginning of pregnancy. Fetuses begin to react to outside sounds at around fourteen weeks. By the end of week thirty five, fetuses can hear low and high frequencies and also differentiate between the two.

Does this impact them in any way?

Absolutely! Ask your partner to monitor fetal movement in accordance with the sound around her and she will tell you that the baby kicks harder when the door slams. Classical music tends to decrease the movements and rock music increases them.

__The sense of sight__: Now, your baby's eyes will be shut for another month or two. And when they open, it will be dark inside the mother's womb. They are still able to do some bit of visual processing. However, this is the least developed sense for your baby when they come out of the womb. Their eyesight is generally blurred as they are born and they are able to see objects that are around 10 inches away from them. This sense is completely developed by around six to nine months.

Your fears and your anxiety: Just like your partner, you too may develop anxiety and fear about the change that you are going to witness in your life. You may sometimes feel the need to turn inwards and withdraw.

Your partner may begin to focus on you more than ever – she has that internal fear (Will he be there for me if I do not lose the extra kilos? Will he continue to love me? Will he love the baby more than me? Will he attend all PTA meetings with me?). Try and read her subtle signs and provide her verbal and non-verbal reassurance that you are in this together.

You may even feel rejected at times because your partner will want to talk about the baby 24 by 7. Don't worry – things will get back to normal soon. This is a good time to talk to your partner about the 'us time.' Let her know that you love the baby as much as you love her and would also want to hear the same from her. Convince her to spend some time, may be a few minutes to start with, with just you and her – let there be no baby conversations during these few minutes. Try and talk about your fears, your anxieties and your dreams – and let her know that she is a part of all these. Let the bonding become stronger than ever.

HOW CAN YOU STAY INVOLVED?

Well, this month you must begin communicating with the baby. This may sound a little absurd, but we all know the importance of good communication. Your unborn baby can hear you and is actually learning from you. Research also proves that fetuses can differentiate between two languages and recognize their native one. Conversing with your unborn baby also helps in developing a bond with the baby.

If you are in military and cannot be a part of this extremely important activity, record a few songs or poems for your baby and ask your wife to play them for your baby, every day at a particular time.

While you want to communicate with the baby often, you must respect your partner. Remember that she has a right to privacy and she may not be completely open to this idea of communication. Let her know the psychological benefits this exercise will have on the child. Did you know that a stubborn breech fetus who loves music can actually change position when they hear music via their mother's abdomen?

Do not whisper to the fetus, speak loud and clear – no, it's not ridiculous and most expectant fathers do it.

Set up a routine – speak to your fetus the same time each day. Try to make it fun. How about gently patting your partner's belly and announcing a prize for a strong kick? It is ridiculous but you will realize the benefits when your baby comes out of the womb – ready to face the world.

Research proves that babies of fathers who regularly communicate with them in the womb:

- Have better attention spans than others
- Hold their heads up sooner
- Cry less at birth
- Mature more quickly
- Sleep better
- Demonstrate advanced level of musical capability
- Develop greater attachment to mom and dad

Sex and pregnancy: Your partner's pregnancy can impact you in a number of ways. Your libido may increase at times. However, some days, the idea of sex can simply put you off.

Don't worry, it's perfectly normal and happening to your partner too.

And the reasons are pretty simple – After around three months, her nausea and fatigue are gone – so both of you feel an increase in sex drive. While you are feeling great at the simple idea of creating life, your partner may be turned on by her new found curves. You may also be experiencing *maieusiophilia*. This is a term used to describe that you may find her body (large breasts and fuller curves) extremely erotic. You may also be experiencing a newfound feeling of closeness towards your partner (She's carrying your baby) and this may manifest itself as increased sexual drive. In case you had experienced a miscarriage earlier, then you would have definitely abstained from sex during the first trimester. The thought of having unprotected sex now can turn you on.

Some men also notice a decreased libido primarily because they do not find the idea of their partner's body transforming from fun to functional really appealing. You may also be scared that sex will hurt the baby and therefore may want to abstain from it.

You must be extremely careful with sex in case your pregnancy has been termed as a 'high risk' pregnancy or your partner has been diagnosed with **placenta previa** (a scenario in which the placenta covers the cervix). Talk to your doctor for guidance if you have had any previous history of miscarriage or any of these conditions.

Try some nonsexual affection such as hugging or simply touching each other.

WHAT ABOUT THE MONTH FIVE HUNGER PANGS?

Not to worry, here are your healthy recipes for month five.

Recipe 1: Mixed berries and coconut smoothie: Blend together ½ cup coconut milk, ½ cup water, ½ cup frozen blueberries, ½ cup frozen raspberries, ½ cup frozen strawberries, 1 tbsp. honey and a handful or fresh mint leaves. Enjoy!

Recipe 2: Monster salad: You will need 1 small bunch each of kale and spinach (chopped), ½ cup Romaine lettuce (chopped), around 10 broccoli florets, 1 diced cucumber, 1 diced carrot, 1 yellow bell pepper, 1 red onion, 6 cherry tomatoes (halved), a handful of blueberries and a handful of walnuts. Take a large bowl and prepare the base of the salad by mixing all the greens. Add the remaining ingredients over the greens now. Consider adding some homemade mango dressing (you know how to make it…yippee!). Enjoy.

Recipe 3: Grilled tuna with celery: You will need 6 Tuna steaks, 2 tbsp. Sesame oil, 2 tbsp. Balsamic vinegar, 1 tsp. grated ginger, 2 cloves of minced garlic, 1 finely sliced green onion and 1 tbsp. lime juice. Mix balsamic vinegar, sesame oil, ginger, garlic, green onion and lime juice. Pour this mixture over the tuna steaks placed in a glass dish. Leave it to marinate in the refrigerator for two hours. After two hours, grill the tuna on medium heat (around three minutes each side). Remove and serve with celery.

Recipe 4: Walnut porridge: Take ½ cup each of raw walnuts, cashews, almonds along with 1 ripe banana, 1 cup milk, 1 tbsp. honey, ½ cup raisins, 1/8 tsp. sea salt and ½ tsp. ground cinnamon. Take a bowl full of lightly salted water and soak the nuts overnight. Rinse and drain the next morning. Pour all ingredients except raisins into a food processor and blend until smooth. Transfer into a saucepan and let it cook on a medium flame for twenty minutes. You can add water, depending on the consistency you want. Remove from heat and sprinkle raisins on the top. Stir well to mix. Ladle into soup bowls and serve warm.

Recipe 5: Baked eggs with roasted pepper: You will need 8 free range eggs, ½ cup finely chopped and roasted red peppers, ½ cup finely chopped and roasted green peppers and ¼ cup grated mozzarella cheese. Preheat the oven to 350 degree F and prepare a large baking dish. Place the peppers in the dish. Crack the eggs over the peppers. Bake in the oven for fifteen minutes or until partly set. Top with mozzarella cheese and bake for another five minutes. Serve warm with some quinoa bread and fresh avocado.

WEEK 21 TO 24: DAD, I LOVE YOU – MORE THAN EVER!

True, this is the time, when the reality of pregnancy has really sunk in, you are now looking forward to your new role and actually reexamining your own relationship with your father. You have never admired and been in awe of your father more than this.

WHAT'S HAPPENING WITH THE BABY?

The baby has still not put on any weight and looks pretty slim. They are also getting covered with a thick, waxy protective coating called **vernix**. Their eyes are beginning to open, they cough at times and get hiccups too. Their movements and senses are getting stronger too – they can hear you, and even respond at times! It is also said the baby's emotions develop during this time.

Girl fetuses develop eggs in their ovaries this month.

WHAT'S HAPPENING WITH HER?

Well, here's some good news! Her moodiness is decreasing now.

However, she still demonstrates forgetfulness and insomnia at times. She still wonders what kind of a mother she would be and needs continues reassurance from you. She also begins to think that she has had enough and now wants to deliver – yes, she is tired and wants to deliver as soon as possible!

Physically, she is a little short of breath as her heart and lungs are working harder than before. There's a little bit of urine leakage during laughing, coughing and sneezing. She is experiencing strong food cravings and sweats more than usual.

The fluid retention in her body increases and may cause compression in various nerves leading to sciatica, carpal tunnel syndrome or simple tingling of nerves.

This is also the period of greatest weight gain and the stretches that she is getting all across are leading to aches and pains all over. Her back hurts and she is often fatigued and dizzy.

You see her face glowing – this is due to the increased blood supply in her body.

WHAT'S HAPPENING WITH YOU?

As you see yourself tied up between various roles – father, husband, partner, son, employee, employer, etc. you begin to reexamine your relationship with your father. You fall in love with your father all over again and are amazed at the manner in which he juggled between various roles.

Now, not all father images are positive. Sometimes, thinking about your relationship with your father may bring about feelings of anger, fear, disgust, etc.

Nevertheless, you will still be reexamining your relationship thinking if this is the kind of role model you want to be for your child.

Always remember that the manner in which your dad parented you will not have an influence on how you want to parent your child. If you feel that your dad was a great father, you would want to replicate some of the things that he did. This could bring back some fond childhood memories. On the other hand, if you do not have great memories about your dad, you are now thinking about ways in which you can be a better father.

This is also the month where you will think about how your baby's life is dependent on you. You will see yourself becoming a better driver and a more responsible person. Suddenly, you will begin to leave for appointments earlier than usual and the traffic signals will have an altogether new meaning. You may even reconsider some of the adventure sports that you may have indulged in earlier. Don't be surprised if you don't want to go for bungee jumping and scuba diving now.

Your partner's overdependence on you may also make you feel trapped. There will be times when you will want to be left alone. Let your partner know about the things that your mind is preoccupied with and talk to her in a non-confrontational manner, always reassuring her that you are there for her but need some alone time to think about various things such as finances, organizing the house, planning the dinner menu, thinking about how you can be a better husband and father, etc.

HOW CAN YOU STAY INVOLVED?

No matter how tensed you are about the reality sinking in, don't let stress take over your excitement. This month, how about some special clothes for yourself and your partner? Customized t-shirts saying *'He's/ She's my baby,' 'Yipee! Three more months to go,' 'Father to be,'* etc. are trendy and can be obtained easily. A water aerobics class with your partner is a great way to build bonding and get some fun into the relationship.

You could even start a scrapbook or photo journal for the baby. Paste pictures of the baby's room (before and after it is ready), your wives belly (the manner in which it is growing with dates e.g. my 1 month old fetus, etc.), baby names, your and your partner's thoughts, etc.

This is also the time when you can begin the process of planning baby announcements and shopping for them too!

Your partner may experience strange cravings such as ice-cream at 2:00am or dirt, chalk, ashes or even the smell of cigarette buds or gasoline. These are absolutely normal. Scientists believe that these absurd cravings are a way of satisfying the body's nutritional needs. For example, there is plenty of calcium in chalk. Your partner may be craving it due to her increased need for calcium.

AND WORK LIFE INTEGRATION TOO!

Most expectant dads begin to bother about quality time with family at this stage. Currently, you are feeling guilty of not spending enough time with your unborn child. Well, you get to spend some time before work, some after work and a little bit on weekends.

Would this be enough once the baby is home?

At this time, you begin to realize that work and family balance are not just a woman's domain. Most working dads today not only strive to achieve that balance but also aim at the perfect work life integration.

No matter how much men may want, only ten percent of dads manage to get more than two weeks off after the birth of their child. The main reason for this is the unpaid family leave that prevents them from spending more time with their new born baby.

I must say, there is a glass ceiling there as well. Just as this glass ceiling prevents women from acquiring the corner office, it prevents men from expressing themselves as equal partners who want to be seriously involved in the upbringing of their children.

My suggestion here is to first talk to your employer or the HR department in your organization about the family leave policies. Tell them how much leave you would need. Claim your family leave – it is your right. Come up with a plan and let your employer know about the benefits of a dad-friendly work environment.

You would also need to keep yourself involved as your child grows up. Think about options there too – these could be working four days a week for ten hours in a day instead of the usual eight hours for five days, or may be doing the split shift (Early morning and late evening) or something like working only three days a week, somewhere closer to your house. Think about whatever works for you in the long term and begin the process of planning now.

Most dads are also thinking about child care options at this time. They begin discussing with their partners on how they would prefer their child to be raised. And sometimes, the agreement is that a loving parent instead of a babysitter has to be there to raise the child. A number of times it is assumed that this loving parent will be the child's mother. What if your partner is earning more than you and has a more stable career? What is she just does not want to stay at home? What if you want to be involved?

The answer to all these questions lies in YOU!

Wait! Wait! Before you flip the pages to read about the next month, I strongly suggest that you give it a thought. Think about the kind of money you would be saving and the quality time that you would be spending with your child. Not to mention, this will strengthen the bond between you, your child and your partner.

ADDRESSING HUNGER PANGS IN MONTH SIX

Here are your month six recipes to treat your partner:

Recipe 1: Tomato and basil juice: Just blend together two tomatoes with a handful of fresh basil leaves. Add a teaspoon of lemon juice into this and drool over.

Recipe 2: Kale and watermelon smoothie: Blend together two cups watermelon (seeded and chopped), half cup kale and a handful of mint leaves. Pour in a large serving mug and enjoy your dinner.

Recipe 3: Spicy and juicy onions to satisfy those pickle cravings: You would need 4 onions (peeled and hollowed), 2 cups chopped broccoli, ¼ cup chopped bell pepper, 2 cubed tomatoes, 1 cup bread crumbs, ½ teaspoon oregano,1/2 cup cubed margarine, ½ cup water, salt and pepper to taste. Hollow the onions by creating a hole in the center. Make sure that you leave the bottom intact. Take a mixing bowl and combine salt, pepper, broccoli, bell pepper, tomatoes, bread crumbs and oregano. Now, fill this mixture into onions. Top with margarine. Garnish with cayenne pepper if you like. Place onions in a slow cooker. Pour ½ cup water around the onions and not over them. Cook covered on low setting for around eight hours. Your juicilicious onions are ready to be eaten!

Recipe 4: Hearty cheesy veggie soup: Mix vegan cream cheese (1 can), vegetable broth (2 cans), chopped carrots (1cup), cubed potatoes (1 cup), chopped onions(1/2) and chopped celery (1 celery stalk) into your slow cooker. Turn the heat setting to low. Cook covered for around nine hours. Add 1 can of baked almond feta cheese. Cook for another half an hour. Stir and season with salt and pepper. Enjoy!

Recipe 5: Chickpeas tomato salad: You would need 1 finely chopped red onion, 2 finely sliced Red chilies, 2 finely chopped Tomatoes, 1 tbsp. extra virgin olive oil, 400 gm. tinned chickpeas, 1 handful of fresh mint, 1 handful of fresh basil and 100 gm feta cheese. Heat the chickpeas and add around three fourth of them into the salad bowl. Mush up the remaining ones and add them too. Add all the other ingredients. Toss, and relish!

CHAPTER FOUR: THE THIRD TRIMESTER

WEEK 25 – WEEK 28: THE NAME GAME AND THE BABY SHOWER!

This is the month where you indulge in the name game. By now, most parents know the sex of their baby and the process of deciding a baby name begins. Those who would like the sex of the baby to be a suspense also begin this activity, just that they keep two lists – one for boy and another for girl.

WHAT'S HAPPENING WITH THE BABY?

Well, your baby is growing now and probably feeling cramped inside the uterus, especially if they have a womb mate. Their eyes are fully open and their iris can react to light and dark. Their lungs are maturing and their skin seems a little less wrinkled (probably due to the fat that they are accumulating). They weigh approximately 2-3 pounds and measure 13-15 inches long. Their brain is still developing and they can even move in rhythm to the music played outside the womb.

WHAT'S HAPPENING WITH HER?

Well, her mood swings are definitely low now as she is getting used to the emotional ups and downs of pregnancy. She is fantasizing about the baby all the time and trying to get things ready for them. She is also concerned about work and worries if she will be able to juggle between various roles – mom, wife, employee, daughter, etc. She is forgetful and secretly fears the process of labor and delivery. *Believe me, she does – even if she does not say so.*

WHAT'S HAPPENING WITH YOU?

Well, now that the idea of fatherhood has completely set it, you too begin to visualize the baby – in your own way though.

Let's do a little exercise here – write down your visualization of the baby and then have your partner write down hers. Although both of you are looking forward to having the baby, the manner in which you visualize is very different.

Most women imagine a baby to be a tiny, cute little person who they will dress up, play with, cuddle, hug and protect from any danger. It's like imagining a fresh from the oven baby with tiny hands and feet along with red lips and pink cheeks.

Men, on the other hand visualize playing catch with their children, holding hands as you walk together on the beach, reading to the child or doing something interactive.

That is the reason why they say *men want children and women want kids*.

For most men, fatherhood is the art of doing stuff, playing with the child, teaching them, mentoring them, helping with homework, etc.

Moms on the other hand can just 'be' mothers. They are mothers due to the physical bond between themselves and their child (When they are in her womb).

This is also evident in the manner in which dads and moms carry their children. Try and observe the manner in which a few new parents carry their babies in front packs. Most moms carry their babies facing in – they are just being moms!

And most dads carry their babies facing out – they are preparing their babies to face the world!

This month you will also begin to speculate about the gender of your unborn baby. You may also begin to call your unborn by a nickname.

Some men prefer a boy to a girl, only because they feel that boys will make great companions at play. If this is the case, please do not let anybody around you know about your preferences. If your child turns out to be the 'wrong' gender (according to you), it will be tough to explain why you had a different preference.

This month you will also be influenced by societal pressures and you will begin to fear.

But you are a strong man, what is there to fear about?

Sure, you are a strong man. But **most strong men also fear labor**. They fear if they will be able to see their partner in so much pain and if both their partner and their baby will be safe. They fear if they will fall apart during labor.

Discuss your fears with your partners. Talk to other dads around and ask them about their experiences. Most dads will tell you that they felt scared, bored, tired, exhilarated, excited or amazed. *And almost all of them would let you know that they would not miss being there for the world!*

HOW CAN YOU STAY INVOLVED?

As your baby is born, the first question that you will hear after 'boy' or a 'girl' would be 'what's the name?'

You need to be prepared to answer that question. Remember, that the name that you choose today is going to stay with the child forever. So, if a name sounds cute today, think about how it will sound when your child goes to college or steps out for a job interview. Try and avoid a rhyming name and think about what the baby's initials would spell. Try and stay away from initials which convert into phrases such as BFF, LOL, STD, HIV, WT, etc.

Think about nicknames too. Would you want a nickname? How would it go with the surname?

Begin the process by making a list of ten girl and ten boy names. Exchange the list with your partner. Strike off the names on her list that you don't like and ask her to do the same for your list. Agree on a common name.

You could even pick up a name book and decide on a name.

Sometimes, you will need to adhere to family customs while picking a name. Keep the above factors in mind before deciding on the final name.

This month, you will also attend your partner's **baby shower**. Earlier, baby showers were considered as 'women only' activities. But now, men participate in baby showers with equal zeal. In fact, you could even plan and organize a baby shower for your partner with the help of a few friends.

The idea behind this is simple – it gives you an opportunity to prepare for your baby's arrival – you get to set up the baby's room through a selection of baby's toys, furniture, accessories, clothes and even cool gadgets. It is a wonderful way to share your excitement with your loved ones.

Now is also the perfect time to look for formats for **birth announcements**. Since you are not sure of the exact time, date and sex of the baby, you would have to wait till the time the actual announcement goes out. However, running for a format would be the last thing that you would want to do once your baby is born.

There are two kinds of formats – an electronic mail format or a hard copy one. Pick up whatever seems nicer and simpler to you and your partner. If you want to use the hard copy print format, then try and get the envelopes ready this month itself.

Most people include the baby's name, time and date of birth, weight, length and the names of the parents on these announcements.

You must send these announcements to your friends and family and also to other business acquaintances who you would like to share the news with.

This is also the perfect time to choose a birthing class for yourself and your partner. Earlier, the focus of birthing classes was limited to providing lessons for a natural birth experience. Now, however, the focus has shifted.

Although, the goal today remains natural childbirth, educating yourself on the entire birthing process – including things like nutrition, exercise and the pain medications that you will need are equally important. The more aware you are, the less you and your partner will fear labor and child birth.

Heard about **Lamaze?**

This is a birthing class that enables you and your partner to appreciate the value of pain and explains definitive steps that you can take to facilitate labor and increase comfort.

Remember, most childbirth classes are exclusively focused on the woman. The women get to socialize and discuss the amount of weight they have gained, the number of times they need to pee during the night or even the color of their vaginal discharge.

Do not be frustrated if you experience this in your birthing class. Instead, go ahead and talk to your instructor about a 'Daddy only get together.' I can assure you that you will be able to indulge in much more meaningful conversations with other expectant dads who will open up to you and talk about similar fears that you are experiencing. They may even recommend certain solutions to the problems that you are anticipating. Talk to your partner before talking to your instructor.

This month is also the perfect time to plan ahead and make some great impact. You have an opportunity to think about how you would like to use the blood from your partner's umbilical cord. This blood is a *rich source of stem cells* that can be used to treat a variety of illnesses such as cancer or leukemia.

You could either donate the cord blood to some other person so that they may benefit. Or you may store it for your family's use.

Doula or no doula?

You and your partner will undergo immense physical and emotional transformation during pregnancy. You are actually in the midst of a trauma as you experience labor. Since you both are under pressure, logically both of you will require support.

They would have taught you so many things in your birthing class – help her breathe, encourage her, rub her legs and back, mop her brow, hold her, reassure her and even feed her ice chips!

So, she has you to help her and take care of her.

But, dad…*you could also use some help!*

The experience of labor is exhausting physically and mentally and you could definitely do with a little bit of a break. This is when a Doula can come for your rescue.

A doula is someone who will be there to provide physical and emotional support to your partner during labor. Using a doula can be expensive. Most doulas charge a flat fee and the American average is around $700. You must check with your insurance company if they would or would not pay for a doula.

You could ask your partner's doctor to recommend a doula. Call them for one or two prenatal visits and then they can stay over for around three hours post child birth.

The presence of a doula can significantly reduce your anxiety levels, and provide you the encouragement to talk to your partner in a more caring and encouraging manner.

HUNGER PANGS IN MONTH SEVEN
Well, here are your month seven recipes:

Recipe 1: Spinach and banana smoothie: Blend two bananas, one cup spinach, ½ cup cacao nibs, ½ cup goji berries and one cup blueberries. You may also use some crushed ice in the blending process. Tastes heavenly, doesn't it?

Recipe 2: Berries and vanilla ice cream: You would need 2 cups of frozen mixed berries (strawberries, raspberries and blueberries), ½ cup coconut milk and 1 tsp. of organic vanilla extract. Pulse the berries in a food processor. Add coconut milk and vanilla extract and pulse once again until a creamy consistency is attained. Freeze for three hours. Serve topped with some dark chocolate shavings.

Recipe 3: Blueberry lime juice: Blend together two limes with a handful of blueberries. Voila, your yummy, colorful snack is ready!

Recipe 4: Garlic flavored potatoes: You would need ½ diced onion, 8 oz. cream cheese, 8 thinly sliced potatoes, 4 cloves of minced garlic, 1 tablespoon parsley and salt and pepper to taste. Put potatoes in the slow cooker. Throw in the other ingredients as well. Set on high. Cook covered for four hours. Enjoy your creamy cheesy garlic flavored potatoes. Delicious, aren't they?

Recipe 5: Sweet potato soup with ginger: You would need 1 pound of sweet potatoes, 1 tsp. extra virgin olive oil, ¼ tsp. Himalayan salt, ¼ freshly cracked black pepper, ½ cup thinly sliced onion, 1 inch piece of minced ginger, 1 tbsp. fresh thyme leaves (chopped), 1 cup fresh orange juice and 2 cups vegetable broth. Preheat the oven to 425 degrees. Peel the sweet potatoes and cut into one inch pieces. Toss these with salt, pepper and olive oil and place on a baking sheet. Bake for around forty-five minutes. Don't forget to toss in between. Now, take a crockpot and cook the onions and ginger in vegetable broth for approximately ten minutes. Keep the flame at a medium-high. Next, throw in the sweet potatoes and let it cook covered on simmer for around half an hour. Add the thyme as well. Blend with a hand blender or puree in batches. You may even store it for use the next day. Just reheat before serving.

WEEK 29 TO WEEK 32: CLEANING THE CLOSETS AND OTHER LAST MINUTE PREPARATIONS

Just a little more time and the baby is going to arrive. Don't be surprised if you or your partner develop an OCD about cleaning the closets and making space for the baby.

WHAT'S HAPPENING WITH THE BABY?

At this time, most babies would have settled in a head down position that they maintain throughout pregnancy. They are getting fat and big – and weigh around five pounds. They are around 18 inches long at this time. The movements are a little less frequent now. However, they are much more powerful and you can actually tell which part of their body is doing the poking. Their sense of hearing has improved so much that they respond to your and your partner's voice differently (you won't know that from the outside). Their tiny heart pumps around 300 gallons of blood every day and they have grown hairy too.

WHAT'S HAPPENING WITH YOUR PARTNER?

You partner has a secret fear now! And it's not just the fear of labor pains…

She fears that her water will break in public. She is also worried if her pregnancy will be normal and if she will be able to survive labor. She is concerned if her baby will be normal and healthy. She wants to know what her baby would look like and is imagining them to be amongst the prettiest babies born on earth. She has begun to feel exceptionally beautiful or ugly and is feeling incredibly special. People are giving her seats in public transport and the store clerks are going out of the way to help her. Strangers are also coming up to her, checking on the health of the baby and even placing their hands on her belly. She likes it sometimes and wants to get over with it at other times.

She is also experiencing the '***nesting***' instinct. As a result, she is making loads of effort to make room for the baby, clear the closets, arrange the cupboards, keep '*unsafe for baby*' items such as cleaning supplies out of sight, organize the baby room, rearranging furniture, childproofing the whole house, etc.

Physically, the frequency of Braxton Hicks contractions has increased. An increased amount of swelling is noticed on her ankles, hands and feet. This is due to the water retention in her body. You will also get worried that she is often short of breath. This is because the baby is taking up the extra space in her body and therefore presses against her internal organs.

She is experiencing stronger and more forceful contractions along with an increased frequency of urination. And then, the general discomfort also reaches its peak.

Her insomnia has increased and so has her fatigue.

WHAT'S HAPPENING WITH YOU?

Well…well….there's no hiding it now. It is obvious and everybody knows it.

Yes, something as private as pregnancy can become public this month. Your partner's increasing belly is actually the center of attraction. You love it when you see people giving her a seat when she travels in public transport or opening the door for her as she goes grocery shopping. You even love the manner in which the store clerk shows concern towards her.

And then suddenly you notice that your partner is chatting with a complete stranger who has approached her with a cute smile saying, 'How sweet! So, when are you due?' and the moment your partner smiles back and responds, they get talking. The next thing your wife may be hearing could be horror stories about a 25 hour labor, an episiotomy that could have damaged the baby's head, a C-section after going through the ordeal of labor for 20 hours, a ten month pregnancy or even anaesthesia that did not work.

You will also notice strangers patting her belly, rubbing it and talking to it as she were some magic lantern or may be a Buddha statue.

Surprisingly, your partner will take it all in her stride. On the contrary, *you may freak out!*

You will begin to think about numerous diseases that could simply spread via touching. You will become more protective about her and even angry about the whole situation. The best option here is to talk to your partner. If she is okay with the situation, let it just be like that. Why fix something that isn't broken? Just try and relax – it happens to all pregnant women. In fact, you may have to deal with a similar situation even after the baby is born – when complete strangers will begin to fondle and play with the baby – and they may not even bother to wash their hands!

This month you may also see yourself spending more time with old friends – in fact even with friends you have not met for years. This is due to the sudden panic that strikes most men during the last two months of pregnancy. They begin to fear that now since their childless days are going to be over soon, they may not get enough time for themselves, their partners or their friends. This may lead to a strange kind of an insecurity and you may try to cover up for things that you anticipate you will miss in the future. These may include eating out, going for movies, plays, reading, gardening or generally hanging out with your buddies.

The powerful 'nesting' instinct also engulfs you and you respond differently than your partner. You try and get the gutters cleaned, get the tyres of your car changes, install safety alarms, and of course learn the art of multi-tasking. If time could permit, both of you would be home with your cleaning gloves on – until the entire house is disinfected.

Your sex life during this time is bound to suffer.

But until last month, things were going fine!

True – the second trimester was the time for increased sexual desire and activity, this month, you may experience strange fears during sex.

What if her orgasm triggers premature labor?

What if you end up harming the baby for your pleasure?

What if she is really uncomfortable?

Her body is changing, will she be okay with the usual sexual position?

Unless your doctor has told you, sex during this time will not pose any risk to your baby or your partner. In fact, some couples use this time as an opportunity to try out some unique and different sexual positions.

HOW CAN YOU STAY INVOLVED?

This month you would also want to plan for the baby's arrival. You really want the baby to arrive in the manner you plan for them to arrive.

Now, you must understand that babies are not particularly great with adhering to these plans. And in most cases the actual process of labor and delivery is very different from what you hoped for. You may hope for a normal vaginal delivery and are fully prepared for it through your birthing classes, antenatal visits, and reading loads of stuff. Your baby, on the other hand may decide not to take that route and the result may be a C-section.

So, what do you do?

Well, I would say go ahead still and create the birth plan. Discuss with your partner, think about how you would want the baby to arrive, talk about your philosophies and write it down.

Next, fold it and keep it in your pocket – this is your cheat sheet if you forget something. Do not show it to anybody else.

The idea is for you and your partner to document the various available options so that you have a clear idea of how to handle stuff – What do you do in case of an emergency? If your partner is unconscious, would you want the doctor to handle or would you want them to first check with you and then do anything? Would you like your partner to take the pain medication right at the beginning of labor or would you prefer to wait? Would you and your partner like to be together throughout labor and delivery? Would she be able to walk during labor? Would you want her to take oxytocin in case she experiences slowdown of labor?

A number of sample birth plans are available on the web. You just have to take a print out and fill in the blanks.

You can choose to discuss this with your doctor too.

You will also want to register for your baby's arrival at the hospital that you have chosen. Most hospitals allow patients to register up to 60 days in advance of the baby's arrival and you don't have to tell them the exact date – because you don't know about it yet! You will just let them know the anticipated date of arrival.

What does it mean for you and your partner?

It means that you will not have to wait at the hospital reception filling out hundreds of forms while your partner is on the wheel chair, screaming and having contractions. Ideally, they must have a room ready for you when you arrive with your partner.

You may also want to check on the hospital's insurance policy.

This month, you and your partner would also spend some time thinking about and finding a competent paediatrician for the baby. A number of family practitioners see babies too. However, most couples want their babies to be seen by a paediatrician, at least during the first one year.

If you have a paediatrician in mind, check on their affiliation with the hospital where your baby will be born. Another important thing is to confirm their night time and weekend availability.

Your partner may want to talk about options to get to the hospital. Would you want to walk (in case the hospital is pretty close) or would you like a friend or relative to take you to the hospital? Driving yourself can be the riskiest of the options as it can lead to several other issues – you may not be able to concentrate since your mind is on your partner and of course, the baby. You may over speed in an effort to reach the hospital soon. Drive only if you are extremely confident that you will reach the hospital on time without any mishappening. The best thing is to arrange for a taxi or a cab.

And what if you have older children?

Plan! Plan! And plan! You must talk to some friends and family members who would be ready to take care of your older children while you are busy in the hospital. Make sure you talk to at least three or four people – you need a plan and then you need a backup plan!

Some last minute things to take care of:

- Stick your doctor's number near the phone and at two or three other prominent places in your house and office.
- Is your car ready? Is the gas tank full? Ensure that an extra pair of keys are placed right near the phone.
- Keep some cash ready for the cab. You never know when you will need one. Place this near the drawer too.
- Check your route to the hospital and make sure that there are no road closures or frequent traffic blockages.
- Make arrangements at work. Labor will come unannounced – always have a tracker ready with how you would like to delegate work and who takes care of your work

once you are on a leave. You don't want phone calls from work when your partner is screaming in pain.

And now let's pack the bags:

Her bag should contain her favorite picture or anything else that she is emotionally attached to and would want during her pregnancy and labor, some soothing music that can help her relax through labor, a bathrobe, a nightgown, some front open shirts, old t shirts that she won't mind getting blood on, a large sports bottle to sip water, some clothes that she could wear when she leaves from the hospital, some nursing bras, old socks or slippers that she won't mind blood on and toiletries including mouthwash, hairbrush, comb, toothpaste, toothbrush, hair ribbons, glasses or contact lenses. Do not carry any jewelry to the hospital.

Your bag should include a few magazines or books that you could read out to your partner if required, some comfortable clothes, a camera with extra batteries and memory card, plenty of cash, some snacks to keep your energy levels up, chargers for your phone, camera or MP3 player, your toiletries including your toothbrush, hairbrush and an extra underwear. You may also need a swimsuit if you plan to get under the shower with your partner.

You must ensure that an infant car seat is properly installed in your car and that you are carrying a washed cute little outfit with legs (just so that the car seat's harness can go between them), diapers and several blankets (stuff depending on the weather) for your baby.

How about stocking up the baby's nursery?

Well, you would need several things in the baby's nursery. Now, people will give you loads of suggestions – some necessary things and some completely unnecessary ones. Here is the list of some of the things that you will definitely need. For all other suggestions that you have received, you can think twice before buying something:

- Baby crib and a crib mattress
- Bassinet
- Changing table
- Side car or co sleeper
- A bath tub
- A baby monitor
- A baby carrier
- Diapers for at least a week (your new born will use around 12-15 in a day)
- An electronic thermometer
- Baby soap and shampoo

- A diaper bag
- A first aid kit
- Nail scissors
- Stroller
- Fitted crib sheets
- Pacifier
- Cotton swabs and alcohol for umbilical cord dressing
- Some formula
- Bottle and breast pump
- Around 10 cute little one piece suits
- Around 10 booties
- 3-4 undershirts
- 3-4 outfits with spate tops and bottoms
- 3-4 sleep sacs
- 6-7 blankets
- 3-4 sweaters
- 3-4 hooded bath towels
- 2 snow or sun hats
- 2 snow suits

Do not invest in a lot of luxury clothes for your little one – they will poop or vomit on them every single day and they will outgrow them too!

Here are some things you will need for your partner:

- Nursing pads
- Milk and vitamins
- Maxi pads
- A comfortable rocking chair
- A nice book detailing how new parents can handle their babies during the first year
- A breastfeeding pillow
- Flowers and chocolates

HUNGRY IN MONTH EIGHT?

Here are some yummy recipes for month eight:

Recipe 1: Peach and strawberry smoothie: Blend together 2 peaches, a cup of strawberries, ½ cup of raspberries and 1 cup almond milk. Enjoy!

Recipe 2: Chocolate pudding: You would need 1 cup coconut milk, ½ tbsp. shredded coconut, 5 tbsp. chia seeds and 2 tbsp. cocoa powder. Add all ingredients in a bowl and mix well. Refrigerate for around eight hours. Remove from the refrigerator and blend till creamy. Refrigerate once again. Serve with a dollop of coconut cream.

*Recipe 3: **Vegan Spanish rice:*** You would need 2 tsp. onion powder, 1 diced green bell pepper, 1 ¾ cup vegetable broth, ½ cup salsa, 2 cups rice, 2 tsp. chili powder, 1 cup tomatoes (diced) and 2 tsp. garlic powder. Just throw everything together in your slow cooker. Mix well to combine. Set on low and cook covered for seven hours. Enjoy the aroma and taste of mouthwatering Spanish rice!

*Recipe 4: **Fluffy almond pancakes:*** Take a mixing bowl and combine ¼ cup coconut flour, ¾ cups almond flour, ½ tsp. baking soda and 1/8 tsp. sea salt. Take another bowl and beat 3 eggs. Next, whisk in ½ cup almond milk along with the flour mixture. Add ½ tsp. vanilla extract and 1/8 cup coconut oil along with ¼ cup honey crystals. Blend until smooth. Now, place the non-stick sauté pan over medium flame and grease with palm shortening. Next, pour ¼ cup of batter on the hot skillet and cook for two minutes on one side. Turn over and cook on the other side for two more minutes. Cook all pancakes one by one. Serve with loads of honey.

*Recipe 5: **Roasted potatoes:*** Preheat your oven to 350 degree F. Peel 1.5 kg. of potatoes and chop them into even sized pieces. Wash the potatoes in cold water and place them in a pan full of water. Add some salt and parboil them (around ten minutes and then drain under cold water). Next, add these potatoes into the baking dish and season with 2 tbsp. olive oil, salt and pepper. Place this dish into the oven and cook for around thirty minutes. Next, squeeze these potatoes with a potato masher. Take a bowl and mix olive oil, 1 bunch of rosemary, 1 bulb crushed garlic and 1 tbsp. red wine vinegar. Add this mixture in the baking dish containing potatoes and give your potatoes a good shake. Cook again in a hot oven for around forty five minutes. Transfer into a plate lined with kitchen paper to drain off the excess oil. Serve warm.

WEEK 33 – WEEK 36: YIPEE…IT'S TIME HONEY!

In just a few weeks from now, you will meet the child you have dreamed about and talked to. You will be a little confused, a little scared, greatly excited, a little jealous…all said and done, you will be eager to meet your baby!

WHAT'S HAPPENING WITH THE BABY?

For most women, this is the last month of pregnancy and your baby is growing at a tremendous rate. They weigh between six to nine pounds before they finally decide to leave the uterus in order to witness the wonders of the outside world. The lanugo and vernix that were covering and protecting them inside the mother's uterus now start to wear off. They are busy preparing themselves for the outside world and therefore spend a lot of time practicing hand clenching, sucking, swallowing, head turning, breathing and blinking.

WHAT'S HAPPENING WITH HER?

This is a difficult time for her. She is tired of being waiting too long, fatigued and frustrated and now she can't wait to see the baby.

While she is excited that she will hold and cuddle her baby in a few weeks, she is also afraid that you won't love her after the baby is born. She has become a little short tempered too. After all, almost everyone is asking her the same question – 'So, when is it due?'

She is also thinking if she will be able to get through labor and is busy making her lists – these are the things that she would like you to take care of before or immediately after the birth of the baby. She is also reviewing the birth plan with you every other day.

Suddenly, she wants to take up an interior decoration course – after all, the baby's room needs to be done to perfection.

Physically, she is experiencing baby movements, although they are not so forceful now. This is because the baby is so cramped inside the uterus that all they can do is to squirm around.

One fine day, the baby's head drops into the pelvis and clears some space off the stomach and lungs. Wow…*she is relieved a bit!*

Overall she is miserable with increased cramps, water retention, swelling, constipation and back ache. She just wants it to be over.

She may have stopped gaining weight and may even lose a pound or so and also loses interest in sex. All she cares about at this moment is the baby.

WHAT'S HAPPENING WITH YOU?

So, it's finally going to be over! In a few weeks, you are going to be a dad!

Well, be prepared. This last month of pregnancy is often the most confusing month for expectant fathers. You may feel super excited at times and totally trapped at other times. Although you now feel ready to be a father, you are also apprehensive if you will be able to do justice to your dual role – being a dad and a husband.

You are now making plans to spend time with the baby and help your partner recuperate. At the same time, you are also worried if you will be able to handle the responsibilities of the house.

"The baby's clothes will need to be washed every day. Will I be able to help her?

Will I remember to load the dishwasher every day? Should I just place a reminder on my cell phone?

Will I be able to balance work and home?

Will she be too weak? Will she be able to guide me through the process of laundry?" – These are just some of the many questions that will be troubling you.

You will feel a strong emotional bond with your partner. However, be prepared as your sex life will completely disappear this month.

You will feel that this is your last chance to spend some quite time with your partner. You may not get this opportunity for the next few months at least. Therefore, you will find yourself spending some quality time with her.

No matter how excited you are, a fear engulfs you – this is the fear of dropping your little baby. You begin to observe how other dads are holding their babies and try to calm yourself thinking that you too will be able to do it.

This month, both you and your partner are increasingly dependent on each other. Although a number of people are offering her advice and support, she needs you to be there for her – almost all the time. You are apprehensive too and therefore want her to understand you.

And here is the funniest part of the story – _you are guilty as hell!_

I find it funny because almost all men begin to feel guilty about what they have put their partners through. They begin to blame themselves and although they want the baby so badly now, they want their partners to be really comfortable – and cannot tolerate the present state. Something that was so desirable at one point in time suddenly converts into guilt.

Don't do that to yourself because your partner realizes that this was her idea too. She also wanted the baby equally badly. Quit torturing yourself and concentrate on the more productive things that you can do for her.

HOW CAN YOU STAY INVOLVED?

This month your partner will be extremely uncomfortable. So, the first thing that you should be doing is to stay near her whenever possible. Reduce your work hours if possible, postpone that long business trip and give away those Friday night outings with friends.

Never leave the house without a phone, she may have to call you in emergency. Also, try and call her 3-4 times a day to check with her on how she is feeling and if she needs anything.

Get her favorite flowers and chocolates every other day.

Even if you are nervous, do not appear to be. She wants to see a calmer version of you – because she is terribly nervous. Try and give her some alone time to rest, read, watch TV – or do whatever she likes doing.

You may also want to review the breathing techniques that you plan to use during actual labor.

Dealing with contingencies – is it true or false labor?

By now, your partner has had enough experience with Braxton Hicks contractions and would probably know when it is time to rush to the hospital.

If you are unsure about whether the contractions that your partner is experiencing are a sign of true or false labor, here are some pointers that can serve as a ready reference:

False labor:

The contractions in false labor are not regular and may get relieved with change in position. A number of women feel relieved as they change position or walk during the Braxton Hicks contractions. These contractions may not get stronger with time and your partner may experience some additional abdominal pain too. Generally, there is no vaginal discharge at this time.

True labor:

The contractions are stronger and regular. The intensity and frequency of contractions increases with time and some blood tinged vaginal discharge is also experienced. Your partner's water may break – that is the amniotic fluid that is discharged as a result of membrane rupture. She may also experience some additional pain in the lower back and this may radiate towards her upper thighs.

HUNGRY IN MONTH NINE?

Well, here are some more recipes to get you going:

Recipe 1: Coconut porridge: You would need 1 mashed banana, 8 free range eggs, ¼ cup almond milk, 2 tbsp. almond butter, 1 cored and chopped apple, 2 tbsp. coconut flakes, ¼ cup pitted cherries and 1 tsp. vanilla essence. Take a bowl and mix all ingredients except apples and cherries. Beat well. Now, stir in the apples in this mixture. Take a nonstick pan and heat the mixture on medium heat. Let it cook into a thick porridge as you stir frequently for twenty minutes. Top with pitted cherries and serve warm.

Recipe 2: Cheesy tortillas: You would need Yukon gold potatoes (1/2 pound), minced fresh chives (2 tbsp.), free range eggs (5), minced garlic (2 cloves), cherry tomatoes (1/2 cup), extra virgin olive oil (1 tsp.) and Manchego cheese (3 tbsp.). Place the potatoes in a pan full of water. Place this pan on stovetop and cook over medium heat for around twenty five minutes. Meanwhile, preheat the oven to 350 degree F. Peel the potatoes and chop into cubes. Now, combine salt, pepper, eggs and chives in a large bowl. Mix well. Heat 1 tbsp. oil in an ovenproof skillet. Add the garlic and potato slices and cook till the potato is golden brown. Add the egg mixture now and heat for around a minute. Press the potato mixture with a spatula and let the egg mixture cook over it for around three minutes. Remove from heat and sprinkle the cheese over it. Bake at 350 degree F for ten minute. Drizzle with olive oil and gently serve the tortillas into a serving dish. Cut into four wedges, top with tomatoes and relish the goodness of cheese and potatoes.

Recipe 3: Roasted cauliflower: You would need cauliflower (1 head – broken into florets), freshly ground pepper (1 tbsp.), sea salt (1 tbsp.), olive oil (1 tbsp.), butter (1 knob), cumin seeds (2 tsp.), coriander seeds (2 tsp.), smashed blanched almonds (a handful), dried red chilies (2) and fresh lemon juice (1 tsp.). Blanch the cauliflower into water for a couple of minutes and leave to steam dry. Preheat oven to 350 degree F. Take a mortar and pestle and bash the chilies, cumin, coriander and almonds. Next, take an oven proof skillet and dry roast this mixture until it gives a nice aroma. Add the cauliflower and cook for five minutes. Transfer into the oven for around twenty five more minutes. Serve hot with quinoa bread.

Recipe 4: Stir fried green beans: You would need 1 lb. green beans, 1 tsp. sesame oil, 1 cup Chinese stir fry paste, 1 tbsp. black bean garlic sauce, ½ cup water and red pepper flakes (to taste). Heat oil in a large saucepan and add the green beans and the red pepper. Stir fry for around five minutes and add water. Cook covered for another four minutes. Increase the heat to high and add the black-bean garlic sauce and the stir fry paste. Cook for around two more minutes or until the liquid has evaporated. Serve warm.

Recipe 5: Chocolate sundae yogurt: You would need fat free Greek yogurt (1/4 cup), natural cacao powder (2 tbsp.), strawberries (1/4 cups) and sliced almonds (2 tbsp.). Add the cacao powder into the yogurt and mix well. Gently stir in the almonds and the strawberries. Your delicious chocolate sundae is ready!

CHAPTER FIVE: LABOR AND CHILDBIRTH
WHAT'S GOING ON WITH HER?

Labor is generally divided into three stages:

- **_Stage one_**: This is the longest stage of labor. In this stage, her uterus will open her cervix in order to enable the baby to descend. During this stage, she would be really scared about the pain she would shortly experience. The contractions in this stage last for around thirty to sixty seconds and come as much as twenty minutes apart. The get longer, closer and stronger over the next few hours. As the contractions keep getting longer and stronger during the second phase of stage one, it is time that you rush to the hospital (if you are not there already). Backache, diarrhea and vaginal bleeding is common during this stage.
- **_Stage two_**: She pushes and delivers your baby. The doctor may encourage her to try a number of different positions. You can even help her using a birthing ball. The back pain is even more intense and a strong stinging sensation is felt by your partner as she delivers the head. This is followed by a sense of relief as the rest of the baby is delivered.
- **_Stage three_**: She pushes and delivers the placenta too! This stage is normally not so important to her because by this time, she begins the process of celebrating your baby's arrival. However, medical practitioners will want to ensure that her placenta is delivered with ease and that she does not experience heavy bleeding.

Sometimes, labor has to be induced through medical intervention. _Your care provider decides to induce labor if her water breaks, or if your baby is overdue._ They may also think about inducing labor in case there is an infection in your uterus or your care provider feels that the baby can now thrive better outside the uterus than inside it.

Labor can be induced in several ways. Whatever methodology your care provider may use, they will need to have her cervix soft and dilated. They might use medicines such as Misoprostol to dilate her cervix. A number of times, these medicines help in inducing labor – this diminishes the need for other labor inducing injections such as oxytocin. Your care provider may call you several hours prior to the time they want to induce labor. This is simply because they want to soften your partner's cervix through Misoprostol.

A number of mechanical techniques are also deployed to induce labor. Sometimes, a catheter with water filled balloon is placed in her uterus. This irritates the uterus and it tries to expel the balloon, thereby softening it further. Your care provider may artificially rupture your partner's water sac. This generally leads to an elevation in the frequency and intensity of uterine contractions. The most commonly practiced method to induce labor is through the injection oxytocin which leads to thinning, softening and dilation of cervix.

She may sometimes require **assisted birth**. This is when her labor fails to normally progress or she develops certain complications. A vacuum extractor or forceps are often used to help with delivery if the baby has descended and your partner's cervix is fully dilated. Your care provider may also use the assisted delivery techniques in case your baby's heart rate is low or your baby is developing certain complications.

A number of times a **C-section** may have to be performed. This is sometimes an elective choice where you and your partner are too frightened to experience labor pain. Your care provider may recommend a C-section if labor is not progressing as it should, your baby is demonstrating an erratic heart rate, your baby is placed in an uncomfortable position, she is carrying multiple pregnancies, her placenta is not healthy and normal, or if she is experiencing some serious health concerns.

WHAT'S HAPPENING WITH YOU?

This is one of the most stressful moments of pregnancy. While your partner experiences intense physical pain, you are experiencing an extreme psychological pain.

The most important thing to remember is that this pain is finite. In a few moments from now, you will be holding God's most beautiful creation – _you will be holding your baby in your arms!_

Another thing to be remembered here is that your partner will forget the pain as she holds the baby. In around 6-8 weeks of childbirth, she would not remember the pain at all and only remember the good things about her pregnancy. (This is probably the only reason women do not resist getting pregnant again).

But dad, it's going to be tough for you! You have watched your partner go through the painful ordeal and just can't get over it. The pain may remain fresh in your mind for the next few years and the thought of forcing your partner into a similar experience once again may frighten you.

HOW CAN YOU STAY INVOLVED?

Try and reach the hospital a few hours in advance and check the room they have allocated to you. Be sure you are aware of the place where extra pillows, blankets, birthing ball, ice chip maker and snacks are located. Check where the nurse call button and shower is located and also find a wheeled stool for yourself. Introduce yourself to the nursing staff and let them know if your partner suffers from any allergies or has some strange fears. Let them know how involved you would like to be. Clarify any doubts that you or your partner may have.

During the process of labor, do everything that you can to make your partner comfortable – backrub, foot massage, rubbing the forehead, wiping the eyebrows – do all that you can! Ask what she wants and make it available for her. If taking a walk seems to be a better idea to her, go along with her.

Ensure that she is hydrated. Feed her with loads of soups and juices in addition to plain water.

Be involved during the active phase of labor too. She needs you most at this time. Remind her to slow her breathing down. Help her relax during the contractions, encouraging her to moan during the contraction and rest in between. Offer cold compresses, ice chips and sips of water. Offer to massage her and keep reminding her that she is doing a great job.

Do whatever your lady wants – don't argue with her, call her names or swear at her.

When you notice a great push, encourage her more. Tell her that is exactly how she should be doing.

If there is a mirror around, encourage her to watch the baby come out.

Don't get shocked when you see your baby. You have been imagining your baby through the nine months and the only images that come to your mind are those chubby little babies that you see in commercials. In reality, babies are generally born covered with a whitish coating called the **vernix**. They can be blue and covered with blood and mucus. They eyes may be closed and back may be full of hair. In addition, they may have a cone shaped head.

And yet.....they are the most beautiful sight in the world!

As you look at the unique person you and your partner created together, you are immensely relieved and overjoyed. The doctors and the nursing staff clean the baby and within a minute of their birth, they are given the **APGAR test**. This is the test that allows the medical staff to judge the condition of your baby.

Right after the delivery, if it is possible, put the baby on her stomach, praise her on how great she was during labor and encourage her to relax.

She has got a new life – **definitely!**

Let's talk about you.

Well, here is a common quote:

"There are three stages in man's life – he believes in Santa Claus, he does not believe in Santa Claus and he is the Santa Claus" - *Anonymous*

So, stage three has finally arrived and you too have got a brand new life, haven't you?

CHAPTER SIX: BABY, IT'S TIME TO GO HOME!

You and your partner have finally made it. You are now the proud owners of a brand new baby. And now begins the testing time.

You have stayed at the hospital for two or three days, your insurance claims are done and now it is time to go home.

This is an exciting time. You and your partner have set up the baby's room, their crib, stocked your home with loads of diapers, baby wipes and bought the cutest outfits on the planet.

The next few weeks will be spent in understanding your baby's physical, emotional and practical needs as you try recover the nine month ordeal. It will take at least a few more weeks for you to return to normal. But it's all worth it! You will enjoy the process as you learn to communicate with your infant and understand their reflexes.

As you take the baby home, you remember the pain that your partner experienced during labor and almost instinctively ask your friends and family to not visit right now. You understand that she may need some rest and the house may not be in a presentable state.

Suddenly, a sleeping baby will become the most precious thing on the planet and you may even turn off the ringer of your phone.

The last but not the least important thing that needs to be mentioned here is that you and your partner, as a parents have made a profound transition into parenthood. You may feel tired at times, but it is extremely important to keep your spirits up. You can eliminate the not so necessary things from your schedule. It is extremely important to be tolerant of yourself and your partner. Both of you are experiencing the joy of parenthood for the first time and mistakes can happen along the way. You must practice forgiveness.

You will need to get some baby skills to eliminate the old school 'mommy does all' philosophy. Spending time regularly with your baby will help you transition from the *'person who takes me to the park'* to *'Daddy'*.

As life begins to settle, you may also fall a prey to ***postpartum depression***.

But I thought that was a woman's thing?

Most studies today are focused on postpartum depression for women, but remember, it is real and guys can get it to. If you experience this, do not panic and seek help.

Understand that from a family of two, you have become a family of three and this third person cannot take care of themselves. So, you and your partner are spending quite a lot of time taking care of this third person. This does not leave both of you with energy to love each other as you used to. In fact, most of your resources are also spent ensuring that your baby gets all that they need in order to make themselves comfortable. So, the gifts that you would earlier shower on each other also automatically decrease.

In fact, everything changes for you – from the manner in which you drive your car to the manner in which you spend your free time (if there is any now).

Your new boss wears a diaper and ensures that you think about them wherever you are!

And here is the strangest part – **YOU LOVE IT!**

You love every single second of this experience and it is so unique that it does not even fade with time.

Congratulations and welcome to Fatherhood…

COPYRIGHT

Made in the USA
Middletown, DE
17 October 2016